WEIGHING

MY

OPTIONS

Suzonne Evans Underwood

WEIGHING MY OPTIONS

Suzonne Evans Underwood

Cover Design by Susan Newman Design, Inc.

Editing and Typography by Patti McKenna

Disclaimer:

CONTENTS

TWAS THE NIGHT BEFORE DIETING

By Suzonne Underwood

"Twas the night before dieting, when all through the house
no creatures were stirring, just me and the mouse;

The cupboards were filled with chips, pies and cookies,
While me and the mouse stuffed both of our tummies;

My family was nestled all snug in their beds,
While visions of chocolate flooded my head;

And I in my rollers and big floppy nightgown,
Had just settled down with a curious frown;

When all in my head all I heard was this chatter,
Was this new lifestyle really going to matter?

Away to the kitchen I flew like a flash,
Tore open the pantry and threw junk in the trash;

The chill from the frig made me wish for some snow,
But whatever the season this stuff had to go;

When, what to my wondering eyes did I see,
But artificial sweeteners to sweeten our tea;

With wisdom and knowledge from this book I had picked,
I knew instinctively it was making us sick;

More eager than Lions as they devour their prey,
I'm sick and I'm tired of our FDA;

I screamed and I shouted and I called them by name,
Oh Sucralose! Oh Saccharin! Oh Acesulfame-K!
Now, Nutri-Sweet, Neotame and Aspartame,
"they claim"!!

Shout it high from the rooftops, from out of the halls,
Throw away! Throw away! Throw away them all!"

Sugar is bad! Here's a good substitute,
We've researched and tested, now skedaddle, now scoot;

We've studied the trials on the mice and their brains,
I laughed and I giggled,
DO THEY THINK WE'RE INSANE?

And then, in a vision, I saw families at home,
Obesity had risen and diseases had grown,

Everyone was scurrying, eating this, drinking that,
With no inclination as to why they were fat;

They were hard working people, educated they seemed,
But trenchermen they were, when they went on a binge;

They couldn't get full, no matter how much they ate,
And their government had fooled them
and used them as bait;

The trials and the data are yet to be seen;
We've now more diseases, now what could this mean;

MSG, High Fructose Corn Syrup and Hydrogenated Oils,
It's all in our grocery aisles, but not in our soils!

The Sodium being added to our foods are insane,
But let's face it people, we're partly to blame;
We bought into the Convenience and Fast Food fads,
Now! Are gone the days of our governing dads?

Person after person got fat and got sick,
They started to read and knew they'd been tricked;

They learned to read Food Labels and what it all meant,
And to their astonishment, oh, the money they'd spent!

The health of their families were seductively hi-jacked,
They knew it was time to take their health back;

They cleaned out their cupboards and started to shop,
They threw out the juices and bottles of pop;

The commodious expansion of space they'd created,
Was doing away with the foods they now hated;

Protein and Fiber, God knew they would need,
It's given in abundance, go eat and take heed;

Good Complex Carbs should be eaten with pleasure,
Fat, Fiber, Protein, they'd eat without measure;

Remember, Drink Your Water,
it takes Pounds out of sight,
"Happy Dieting to all, and to all a Good-Bite!"

INTRODUCTION

Perhaps, the single most common goal among adults is to lose weight. While that goal might be widespread, 50 pounds, 20, 10, or just enough to zip your jeans without lying down, each pound can seem like a lead weight that refuses to let go.

It seems that there are just as many ways to lose weight as there are people who wish they could. There are packaged dinners from different weight loss programs, exercise franchises, pills which promise to burn fat, suppress the appetite and increase metabolism, and let's not forget the diets. Dieters can choose from protein diets, low-fat or low-carb diets, the South Beach diet and Adkins diet, as well as the good old standbys, like the grapefruit diet.

The problem is those diets don't work by themselves. Sure, we can lose weight if we follow them, but whatever caused us to gain weight in the first place eventually comes back and interrupts our diet. As a result, we slow down our progress or, worse yet, fall off our weight-loss regimen completely. Usually, we gain back most or all of the weight we lost, and sometimes more.

I'm not an expert, but I have found something that works and works well. It's not a diet plan you can follow step by step, measuring grams of fat or carbs, but it is a plan that has been proven to be successful in long-term weight loss. The secret of this plan is not specifically the foods involved, but that it contains one ingredient most diets don't—feeding your mind. By feeding your mind, I mean replenishing your self-esteem, having a positive attitude, finding motivation and the determination that you are ready to make a lifestyle change and that you have the confidence that you can, no—you will, succeed.

This book will show you how to lose weight the physical way, but it will also show you how to lose weight the mental way. By following the steps in this book, I lost 15 pounds in one month. Perhaps the greatest achievement wasn't what I lost, but what I gained—a better understanding of why I gained weight and the attitude and mindset to do something about it. I've found that those things are so important in weight loss that I've made them the first parts of this book. Outer beauty is important to most of us, but it's the inner beauty and confidence that will make it happen.

The purpose of this book is to show you how you can undergo a body makeover, while creating a frame of mind that supports you along the way. Most of the time, it is our mind that defeats our purpose by creating doubt and discouragement. I'm going to show you how to change that once and for all so you can create an image that is worthy of the wonderful person that you are.

Let's get started and learn what you can do right now, today, to create a better tomorrow for your body, your mind, and your life.

SECTION ONE:

THE

PREPARATION

Chapter One

THE ONE THING EVERY DIET SHOULD CONTAIN: A CHECKUP

This book is intended to provide motivation and weight-loss tips and suggestions which can be incorporated into almost anyone's life. I've used the ideas and concepts in this book, and am glad to say that I've had good results. You won't find a specific diet plan within these pages, but rather, you'll find ways to change your eating habits and lifestyle, along with suggestions that worked for me. I won't devise a diet plan for you because everyone's individual needs are different. Every _body_ is different. What you will find within these pages are real suggestions which you can use in your own diet plan to promote weight loss that is less limiting and costly than many diet plans marketed today.

I hope you'll find that my weight-loss strategy is less restrictive and more flexible than most. It's not intended to be a diet you follow by the letter, but a change in your eating habits and lifestyle which you adapt to your specific needs. You are in total control of the foods you eat, when and how often you eat, and the options you wish to integrate into your own diet plan.

But before you get started, I highly encourage anyone considering a weight-loss program or a change in their eating habits to consult with a physician before they begin their journey. A doctor is knowledgeable of your body's needs and requirements and is best suited to help you devise a weight-loss program for your body. In addition, people with health issues should always seek a doctor's approval before making any changes in their eating habits to ensure their body is getting proper nutrition and a balanced diet which addresses those needs. A physician can also provide you with additional information or tools which will make sure your weight-loss plan is a safer and easier one.

Once you've visited your doctor and received his or her approval, I hope the information shared in this book will help you achieve your goals and keep you motivated to make healthy choices in your diet and your lifestyle. These suggestions have been successful in making my life healthier and happier. I encourage you to use or adapt the ones which are best suited for you. In dieting, as in everything, you have choices. By weighing all of your options and finding what works for you, you will make your journey toward becoming thinner and healthier an easier one.

Chapter Two

DON'T WAIT UNTIL YOU LOSE WEIGHT: BECOME THIN NOW!

When we gain weight, it shows on the outside, increasing our waist line, hips, and thighs. The effects of those extra pounds are evident on our physical appearance, but it's just as true that their impact is more profound on our inner thoughts, opinions, and beliefs. Our physical image influences the mental image we have of ourselves, and both of these play a role in our overall health. Is the mind stronger than the body, or vice versa? Which one will help us most in our battle to lose weight?

The answer to that question is as unique to each person as they are. Regardless of which is stronger, it's become apparent to me in my quest to lose weight that success will only happen if I have the mental determination and motivation to make it happen. We can all desire to look different, be different, and create a healthier lifestyle, but until we change our attitude, we can't change our appearance.

For example, some people put things off, dreaming of all the things they'll do after they lose weight. They'll get a new hairstyle, buy a new wardrobe (or at least a few must-have pieces), start an exercise program or a new hobby, or participate in groups or activities that interest them. But, it's all based on whether or not they lose weight. Why? Why does everything revolve around that one factor—our body weight? Why do any attempts to improve other areas of our life depend on where the needle rests on the bathroom scale?

It's like which comes first, the chicken or the egg? Is it necessary for us to first lose weight, then create the person we want to be and the life we want to live, or should we begin with an attitude and mental makeover which will help us achieve our weight loss goals? Maybe that question can best be answered by the old adage of the person who is contemplating going back to school to earn a degree. Arguing that it will take 4 years of schooling and that they will be 48 (or whatever age) when they graduate, they dismiss the idea. However, that reasoning is often countered with the statement, "You're still going to be 48 in 4 years. Would you rather be 48 with that degree or without that degree?"

Apply that reasoning to all of the things you put off or dismiss, saying that you'll do that once you lose weight. What happens if you don't lose weight? You'll never undertake any of those things or enjoy any of those new experiences? Why not start now? What's holding you back besides a few pounds?

Losing weight is a challenge and one that won't happen overnight. As a matter of fact, it might take many nights before you begin to see real results in the mirror. But, there are things you can do today which will not only help you to lose weight, but which will improve your attitude, build your self-esteem and propel your motivation to create change. The desire and motivation for change starts with your mind. Without it, there would be no yearning to be slimmer and trimmer. So, I propose that while you have that desire and motivation, you use it to make immediate changes that will fuel your other desires along the way.

First, in order to be a thin person, you don't have to be thin. Really. Becoming thin is not only about dieting and shedding pounds; it's about feeling like a thin person, acting like a thin person, and thinking like a thin person. It's about believing that you can be a thin person and then living life like you already are!

Are you waiting to lose weight before you buy a new wardrobe? Why wait? What's wrong with looking the best you can today? Go ahead, try on new clothes and styles that fit your body just as it is. Dressing in clothing that is attractive and enhances your shape will not only make you look better, but it will also make you feel better. It will motivate you to stay on your diet so you can dress and look the way you want when you are slender. But, too many of us hold the mindset that we have to lose weight first, and worry about the wardrobe when we've downsized our body. That's where we're so very wrong. We need to appreciate our body right now, at this very minute, and make ourselves look as attractive and appealing as we can today. It might take two or three months to lose a dress size—should you have to wait two or three months to look good and feel good about the way you look?

Dress like a thin person, act like a thin person, and think like a thin person. Picture what your life will be like when you are thin, then go ahead and start living it! Life is far too short and uncertain to waste one single minute waiting to experience it to its fullest. Don't shy away because you need to lose weight. If someone wants to take your picture, stand tall, proud, and thin, and smile with confidence! Are you waiting to begin an exercise program until you've lost 15 pounds? Pretend you've already met your goal, and start taking brisk walks, following an exercise routine, or join a gym. Not only will you feel more energized and become healthier, but you'll speed up your weight loss in the process.

Make your life a thin routine. Finish this sentence, "When I lose weight, I'll …" Envision your day from the moment you awaken to the time you go to bed at night. Will your routine change once you've lost weight? If so, how? Now, write that schedule down. Get in the routine *before* you lose weight, not after! Wake up at the same time every day, read your daily affirmation or spend some quiet time each morning in God's word, exercise first thing (even if you dread it), shower, then get ready for your day. Fix your hair in that new style, you know, that style you've put off getting until you've lost weight, then put on your makeup, take a look in the mirror and tell yourself how great you are and how good you look!

Begin today to make sure your routine includes your diet and the foods you need to be eating to become thin. Remember, breakfast is the most important meal of your day. How you envision and start your day will have a huge impact on how the rest of your day goes. When you're thin, will you eat a donut for breakfast or will you choose yogurt or fresh fruit? Eat the way a thin person eats! Log your breakfast and your snacks throughout the day, becoming conscious of everything that goes into your mouth—you might just be surprised that you're eating more than you thought! Become conscious of habits which do not support your goal to be thin, and you'll be more attentive to changing them.

Plan your day and plan your life while you're becoming thin. Start with your weekly grocery shopping. Plan your weekly menus. It's much easier to stay on a plan when you're cooking the same for the entire family. I've found that it's so much easier to stay on a diet when I make a grocery list, making sure that I remember to purchase "thin" and healthy foods which will satisfy my tendency to snack throughout the day. Never go grocery shopping hungry! I even go one step further, and when I come home from the store, I package my snacks in pre-measured containers or snack bags, if they're not individually wrapped, so I can grab or throw them in my purse whenever I feel a hunger craving coming on. It eliminates the temptation to choose a less healthy and more fattening alternative! Also, to keep my metabolism running at full capacity, I make it a rule of thumb to eat three healthy meals a day with two high fiber and protein snacks. I always eat every 2-1/2 to 3 hours. No more, no less. And I never eat after 8 pm.

When you're done planning your "week as a thin person," plan your life. How will your life be different once you've lost weight? Will you be more active? Will you take up a hobby, like tennis, golfing, swimming, skiing, hiking, jogging, painting, or writing? Why not start now? The things you enjoy or desire in life are too important to put on a backburner, keeping them out of arm's length until you've lost weight. Indulge yourself and pursue those activities today! Go to your community college and register for an art class, join an exercise group, buy yourself a pair of skis or hiking boots and begin to pursue enjoyment in your life.

You are the most important person in your life. Don't be a prisoner to your weight. Today is here; why not find pleasure and even pride in it? Do something to build your confidence, boost your self-esteem and make real strides toward the person you want to be. When you invest in yourself, you build positive thoughts and opinions that you are worth the time and the investment, not only to lose weight, but to embark on a new lifestyle that will bring you immense satisfaction, regardless of your weight.

Tomorrow will come, but if you keep doing what you've always done, you'll keep getting the same results you've always gotten. Overweight and miserable! Tell yourself every morning that just for today, you are going to live an abundant life, enjoying the activities and pursuits you've put off for too long. Remind yourself that you are, indeed, worthy and take pride in the person you are at this moment. Too many people are guilty of waiting for certain events to happen or to accomplish certain things before they take care of themselves and take pride in the person they are. You are unique; there's nobody in the world just like you. What better time than today to be the best person you can possibly be? Our tomorrows are uncertain, and all we really have is today. Psalm 118:24 says, "This is the day which the Lord hath made, we will rejoice and be glad in it!"

Chapter Three

VISUALIZE YOUR SUCCESS

Have you caught yourself daydreaming, envisioning a more slender you down the road? Take advantage of it and use those visualizations to propel you toward your goal!

The process of becoming thin is often about thinking thin. It's living like you're thin, acting like you're thin, and eating like you're already thin. That's one reason why this diet works for me—because from the beginning, I'm eating a diet which will be the very same after I've met my goal. I'm not on a diet first, then on a maintenance program. It's a lifestyle change based on the weight I desire to be, not the weight I am.

So, while I'm making wise food choices and eating like a thin person, I've found that it's helpful to visualize my life as a thin person. What will I look like? Will my wardrobe change? Do I see myself on a beach, running a marathon, on a golf course, or in a dance class? Some might call this daydreaming, but in reality, it's visualization, which is a very powerful motivator.

Visualization can be done with more than the mind, though. Having difficulty creating the thinner image you'll be when you've accomplished your weight-loss goal? Pull out an old photograph of yourself at a time when you were slender. Get on the computer and edit a picture, putting your face on another person's body. You'll begin to be able to imagine yourself pounds lighter immediately!

The process of visualizing can include more than visions of yourself. Is one of your goals to lose enough weight so you can fit into that little black dress that you love, but can no longer wear? If so, take the dress out of hibernation and hang it where you'll see it everyday. It will inspire you to stay focused until the day you proudly pull the zipper up with ease.

The secret of using visualization is that it helps you create a 'can do' attitude. By seeing the results before they actually happen, you create the mindset of success. It instills the belief that you can and will become slimmer and healthier, while removing doubt.

I also suggest that you remove some things from your vision. Is there a dessert cookbook on the shelf? Tuck it away while you're dieting to remove any temptations. Don't buy magazines with fancy desserts on the cover; choose instead to read inspirational books or magazines. Spend an hour framing your favorite motivational saying and hang it where you can see it often.

As you lose weight and your body downsizes, your clothes will become too big! That's one of our favorite parts of dieting—when we can actually tell that it's working! When that happens, remove those old clothes so they don't serve as an unconscious reminder that they're still there—just in case you should need them. To be a thin person, remember, that you have to live like a thin person and look like a thin person, in your mind, as well as in the mirror.

Chapter Four

KEEP IT POSITIVE

Diets have historically been given a bad rap. They've been dreaded, bemoaned, and the victim of many a complainer. Diets have been short-lived, put off, and ditched. If a diet is supposed to actually be good for us, why is it that we hate them so much?

Maybe it's our outlook. A negative perception can create negative results. If we start a diet with the belief that we will ultimately fail, we will. If we view a diet as temporary, it won't last long at all.

How do we counter that negativity? By being positive! A diet doesn't have to be your enemy—it can be your friend! Simply stated, a diet doesn't have to be a bad thing if you view it as a positive component in your overall goals for self improvement.

So, why not think of a diet in a positive manner? Instead of saying "I've got to go on a diet," try, "I get to start a new lifestyle." That's a switch, isn't it? What happens when you change the wording? You change your perspective, removing negativity from the event.

Because I know that my new lifestyle is a positive step toward looking and feeling better, I like to think of it as my friend. It's a companion I keep with me at all times, reminding me to treat my body better and give it food and nutrition which will help it perform and feel better.

Yet, I do know that it's easy to get discouraged. There are times when the weight doesn't come off as quickly as we want or when we lose some of the initial momentum and motivation that inspired us in the first place. That's when I count on my affirmations to reinforce and support my goals.

Affirmations are positive statements we make as a means of reinforcement, encouragement, and most of all, to cement our belief in our goals. They are powerful ways to think thin while we're becoming thin.

Affirming your goals and your belief that you'll meet them will help you overcome one of the biggest obstacles in losing weight—negativity. Negativity creates failure, but positive thinking promotes success. That's why affirmations are always worded in a positive manner, and they're purposely worded in such a way that they declare success, even before it's achieved.

When you're making your own affirmations, make sure you believe them. Make them your own, and own them. Your affirmations won't be the same as anyone else's because they hold your beliefs, your motivations, and your emotional triggers. There should be no room for doubt in your affirmations—so remove words like "can" and replace them with words like "am." For instance, instead of saying, "I can lose ten pounds," try saying, "I am losing ten pounds." The former says that it's possible, but the latter says you're already achieving it.

Here are several examples of affirmations you can use to help you lose weight and become healthier. Feel free to choose any or all of them or make your own!

"I am becoming healthier every day."

"I am in the process of losing weight and become fit."

"I feel lighter each and every day."

"Today, I am eating foods which are good for me."

"I am thinner and happier."

"I am more energetic each and every day."

"I enjoy eating foods which are healthy, natural, and wholesome."

"I enjoy spending my time enjoying new activities."

Once you've written the affirmations which resonate with your goal, beliefs, and emotions, it's time to let them make a positive impact on your life. Write them down and put them where you'll see them as soon as you wake up. Post them on the refrigerator door, marquee them along your computer's screen saver, and place a copy on your bathroom mirror where you'll see them throughout the day.

But for affirmations to be truly effective, you must say them. Repeat your affirmations out loud every morning and every night. Say them with conviction, removing any and all doubt from your voice, your tone, and your mind. When you do, your affirmation becomes a part of you and your weight-loss plan. It's an ingredient some of the most successful people in the world have used to meet their goals, and it might possibly be the most important thing you can do to inspire and motivate you toward your goal. Belief isn't a little thing. It's everything!

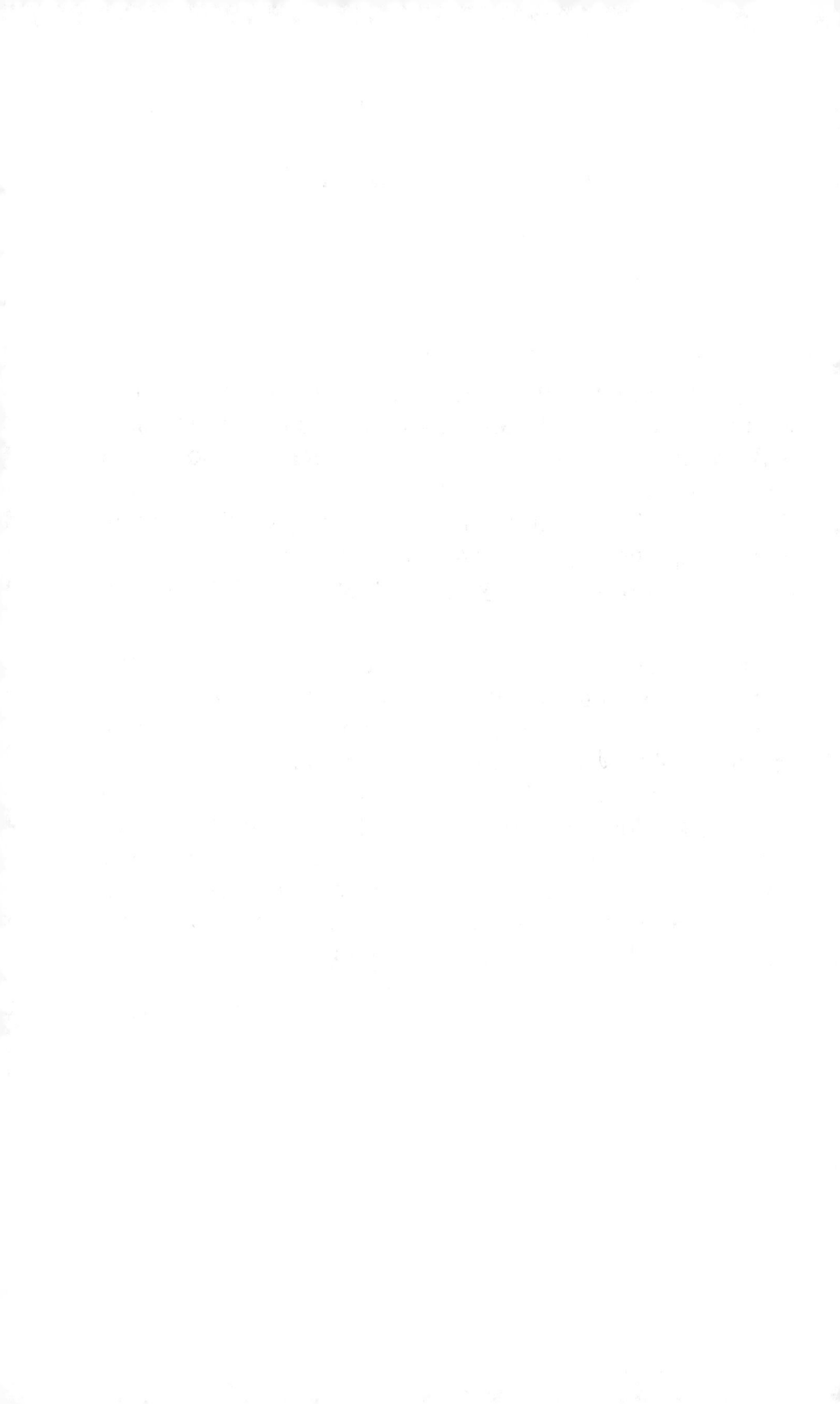

Chapter Five

TO LOSE WEIGHT,
FIND OUT WHY YOU GAINED IT!

Okay, you're packing a few extra pounds and have decided it's time to lose some weight. Good for you! But, before you get started, I'm going to ask you to take a trip back in time. Your time capsule is going to help you to lose weight, and it will also help you keep it off.

Does that sound backwards to you? Why are we looking back when we need to move forward? Well, we have to go back in time to determine just what it was that caused you to put on that weight in the first place. What did you do, or not do, that tipped the needle of that scale in the wrong direction?

Has Father Time been friendly to you? I'm not talking about aging, though, that catches up with us, too! I'm referring rather to how your lifestyle and eating habits may have changed throughout the years. When we were younger, it sure seemed like our body could take abuse a little easier, and Mother Nature was a little kinder, too! We could eat what we wanted, when we wanted, and as much as we wanted, and the mirror was still our friend. What happened?

At what point did you notice that you weren't able to maintain your weight as easily? When did it take a couple more inches of the measuring tape to circle your waist than it had before? Was it when you graduated from high school or was it the freshman 15—you know, the initial 10 or 15 pounds they say college freshmen gain from eating food out of a vending machine or from fast food restaurants? Maybe, it was when you got a desk job or after you had a child or three? These are all reasons why we gain weight, and they'll open your eyes to what you need to do to counter it.

When I did my internal time research, I found out something I wasn't aware of before. I was bored—plain and simple, I hit a stage of boredom in my life and started to feed it. Having little or nothing to do allows for a lot of time to eat, take my word for it! I was filling my stomach while I was filling my time, and one day, it hit me. Based on my waist line, I obviously had far too much time on my hands.

Boredom is simply a lack of anything exciting to do with your day—anything, other than the usual run of the mill daily duties that go along with raising a family and meeting demands. Sure, with a husband, kids and a house, I had things to do, but they weren't things that excited me. It was repetitious household chores and obligations, which surely didn't raise my excitement meter. I should point out right away that depression and boredom aren't the same. Depression is a state of mind, and sometimes, it can be more than a temporary state. In addition, depression can be the result of or cause other physical or emotional problems, so I encourage anyone who is suffering from depression to see their physician for diagnosis and/or treatment.

That said, I had to figure out how to keep boredom at bay. I had to find a way to stay busy in order to break my habit of using food to fill that void. And, that's just where the change began. Just what was I going to do? I wasn't passionate about exercising, but it was obvious that I had to take some action and create some new activity in my life. The bad part was I'd gotten into a rut—a daily routine of doing the same old, same old, day in and day out. I was so restless!

As soon as I realized what caused my weight gain, I had to figure out how to become "unbored." I had to find something that I was passionate about that diverted my mind and my body enough that I'd forget about eating. While I've always been very actively involved in my children's life, schools, community, and church, that wasn't enough. After all, I was already doing that, and I was still restless. Have you ever heard the saying "you can be in a room with a large crowd of people and still be lonely"? You can be bored when you have things to do and places to go. What I needed wasn't something to do, but rather something I was passionate about doing— something new, exciting, and fresh. Above all, I wanted that something to be for me for a change. I've always happily invested my time toward helping other people and causes, but I knew that whatever I chose had to be personal. It had to fit my mind, body, interests, and lifestyle and enhance them as much as possible.

I found my passion through writing and expression. I'd always wanted to write, but it was something that I placed on the backburner because I was busy being a wife and a mother first. With a husband practicing law, one child graduating high school and about to leave for college, and another in elementary school and other extra-curricular activities, I finally had some time on my hands. I dusted off that old interest and decided to see where it would take me. First, I had to figure out just what to write about, which was easy for me since I'm passionate about so many topics. If writing was my passion, maybe the answer was just as clear—I should write about what I'm passionate about! I was onto something! I'm also studying interior design in my spare time. Everyone has something they're passionate about!

My point is, you have to know what factors contributed to your weight gain in order to turn it around. Then, you have to remove yourself from those things and find something you're passionate enough about so you don't miss them. It has to be big enough to create more than a weight change—it has to create a lifestyle change so you don't fall back into the old habits and routines which caused you to put on weight. Throw yourself into it 120 percent if you have to, just do it! It will be as effective, if not more effective, than any diet or weight loss program you'll ever invest in. As Dr. Phil would say, "You have to get excited about your life!"

Taking a glance down memory lane, I can see how easy it was for me to get into a rut without even knowing it. I wasn't blind to the fact that I'd grown a little here and there. After all, the mirror doesn't lie and neither do tight clothes. But, there was always tomorrow. There was always an excuse to stay right where I was just for today; I could worry about my weight tomorrow. My trip down memory lane reminded me of how many times I'd promised myself to begin a new lifestyle on Monday. Then, Monday would come, and before I knew it, I was committing that promise to next Monday, and so on. In the end, I hadn't taken a single step toward losing weight or becoming healthier and more fit. I'd just gotten very good at making (and breaking) promises to myself to do something about it. Not only had I gotten into a rut, my life had become robotic. I was going through the daily motions without emotions of any kind, except boredom.

It took more drastic measures than knowing that I needed to lose weight or even wanting very badly to do so.

My quest to become thinner didn't actually take root until I took ACTION—mentally creating a change in my life so I could physically create a change in my size. It was one of the best things I could have done. While I'm busy writing, juggling deadlines, reviewing graphic designs, illustrations, working on websites, learning about the marketing world of book publishing, etc., I'm learning and keeping myself out of the kitchen. For once, my body is shrinking and my mind is expanding. Some days, the excitement I feel about my life now is overwhelming, to say the least! The question you need to answer is: What will it take to keep you out of the kitchen? What one thing (or several) can you change in your life which will be big enough to have an effect on your jean size?

If your job is sedentary and that's what contributed to your weight gain, how can you change it? Should you exercise, or should you embark on physical activities which excite you, like tennis or skiing? Figure out what caused your weight gain, then find something just as significant to balance it out. Not only will you lessen your burden, but you'll also lighten your load.

Chapter Six

LOVE YOURSELF

Shedding pounds means shedding old attitudes. Sadly, many overweight people have a negative opinion of themselves. They feel like they have less to contribute to others, and sometimes they don't feel like they're worthy of living a rich and rewarding life. Overweight people tend to harbor shame for the way they look; as a result, they are overly critical of their appearance and have low self-esteem.

Why? I know that I'm the same person I was in my more slender days. Yet, my disapproval of my weight created a different viewpoint of the person I'd become. Sure, I thought of myself as a loving mother and wife, a friend, and a member of the community, but I became aware of the fact that my opinion of myself was also based on my weight. As someone who is usually self confident and assured, I knew that it was time for me to do something about changing my opinion of myself and regaining my confidence in not only my abilities, but in my whole self. I no longer wished to feel self conscious about my weight and decided to do something about it.

As children, we love ourselves. We feel comfortable in our own skin, regardless of what we may look like. We aren't self conscious or worried about what other people think of us. Then, we become adolescents and are subjected to criticisms and a desire to be accepted by others. For those who are overweight, that can be a difficult time.

Our negative opinions of ourselves get in the way of our positive progress. Regardless of what we attempt to accomplish, a negative attitude or opinion will hinder or halt any steps we make toward positive change. I think that opinions and attitudes make a huge difference in life, so I have a saying that I repeat to myself whenever I catch my inner voice becoming critical: "If I want to better myself, I must think better of myself." Not only is it catchy and easy to remember, but it's true!

Every transformation or change we attempt to make in ourselves must start with our mind. That's where the desire to change originated, in this instance to lose weight, and it's where we have total control over whether or not we'll actually follow through. Some people call it mind over matter, but I know that our thoughts are where we begin and they also determine where we'll end.

Regardless of how much weight you want to lose or why you want to lose, your self-esteem and confidence are going to determine your results. I've found that it's important to have self-esteem and confidence *before* I lose weight, rather than working on building those things after I lose weight. Again, there's no reason to hold off on improving your mind and your body, waiting to lose weight first. The mind comes before everything else. Because of that, my weight loss plan integrates daily affirmations, supporting my progress and my goals. They keep me motivated and inspired, and they also help my mind believe what my body can achieve.

The next time you begin to feel discouraged or you "cheat" just a little, don't let it be the end of your weight loss plan! Let it be the beginning. Find something to motivate you, whether it's a photograph of a newer, thinner you, or taking a brisk walk. Get your mind off food completely and don't dwell on your diet or your weight. Physical activity will help, and so will removing yourself completely from the kitchen (or even the house) where you won't have access to food. Then, do something that invigorates your mind or your body to get yourself back on track. It will help you control your cravings while giving you a chance to turn your thoughts to something more interesting than your next snack or meal. Everyone has something that they truly love to do or be engaged in. Find what that something is for you and pour yourself into it fully and completely. Learn to cross stitch, sew, needlepoint or paint. A new hobby just might be the appetite suppressant you've been searching for all this time!

Chapter Seven

IT'S ALL ABOUT YOU,
BUT SOMETIMES IT'S ABOUT
EVERYONE ELSE, TOO!

While it's critical that you create a self image that supports the person you want to be and the life you want to create, that can be a very solitary experience. To create change in your life, you also need to create new experiences, meet new people, and embark on new causes. Those things will make your life richer and more rewarding. They'll give you a greater purpose, as well as keep your mind off the fact that you're dieting. Keeping busy is a great way to divert attention from things you want to avoid and helps to increase physical activity, curbing any tendency to be sedentary, which is often one of the reasons we gain weight as we grow older.

Once you've decided to lose weight, you've made a decision to care for yourself. You've consciously decided that you want a healthier life, a better life. Congratulations! This is also a great time to reach out to others, improving your life by improving the lives of other people in your community. Do you have a favorite charity that could use your help? Volunteer to help in their next fundraiser, making calls or using your specific talents and skills where they're needed. Do you enjoy spending time with people who are less fortunate than you? You might want to spend time visiting children in your local hospital or seniors in a nursing home. These are all things which will boost your self esteem and bring you a sense of pride in your contribution. They will make you feel worthy and remind you that you are appreciated just the way you are. Again, we're reinforcing the fact that the quality of your life doesn't hinge entirely on your weight. You have qualities, talents, and gifts to share with the world, and it would be a shame to wait until you've done x, y, or z to benefit from them.

Shed your self-consciousness and reach out to the world as if you were already thin. Don't step back and wait in the wings, becoming an observer in life. Be a participant! Make friends and join groups where you'll find that your opinions and your company are appreciated, ridding yourself of any negative thoughts you may have developed about yourself because of your size along the way. Negativity is a certain way to deter success, and it's something we'll discuss in much greater detail. But for now, know that positive actions create positive results. Using your talents and time toward positive causes will fuel your desire to create positive results in all aspects of your life. It's a very powerful and rewarding experience that will boost your pride and confidence levels to new heights.

I also encourage you to find a friend or a group who will support you in your weight loss goals. Tell your spouse, your child, your best friend, or your sister what you're trying to do. Be sure to choose an individual who is positive and is a cheerleader, someone who will celebrate your milestones with you and provide you with the necessary support and encouragement you'll need to accomplish them. Life isn't a solitary event—it's about being with people and sharing with them. Share your goals, and ask your weight loss supporter to keep you on track and motivated. Most people will be flattered that you think so highly of them and will be happy to be a part of your success.

There's one other person that I want you to address, and that's yourself. Get rid of your monkey mind! Stifle that little voice inside you that reminds you that you've tried to lose weight before and it didn't work. Today is a new day! This is all about you and your quest for self improvement, but it's also about the people in your life. In order to be successful, surround yourself with people who support you and steer clear of anyone who tries to discourage you, even if that person is the doubt that exists within yourself.

You can control your life, starting today. Believe that you are worthy, take pride in the way you look and the things you do. Create the mindset of a winner, and then act like one. When you do, amazing things will happen.

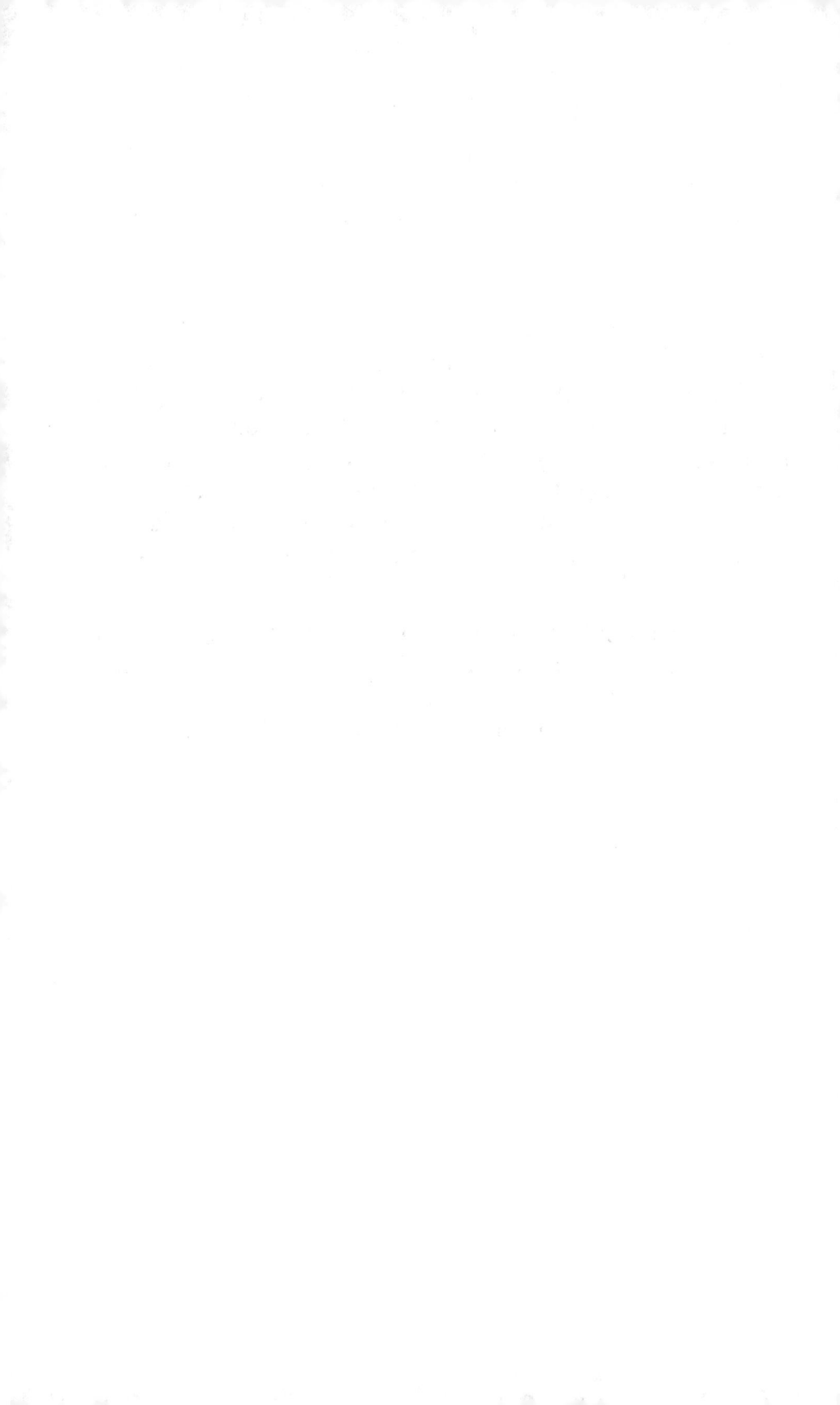

Chapter Eight

IT'S A FAMILY AFFAIR

Admit it. You didn't gain weight alone—you had other people helping you. As a matter of fact, they might have been the reason why you gained weight in the first place. Most likely, those people are the people you love the most, the people you live with—your family.

I'm not accusing your spouse or kids of force feeding you cookies, cake, ice cream, and potato chips! No, this isn't the blame game, but I am saying that it's hard to diet alone. Nobody spoon fed you the food that went from your lips to your hips, but the lifestyle and eating habits of the people you live with are contagious! Think about it. You cook for your family, often giving them what they need and want, knowing that you can't deprive them of the foods they like because you want to lose weight, right? That wouldn't be fair. So, as long as you cooked it and it's hot and ready, you eat it, too. This is also true of snacks— you might not be hungry at all, but when it's time to give your kids a snack, you also grab a cookie or two for yourself.

We pick up the same habits as the people around us, and that's also true when it comes to what we eat and when we eat. We fall into the same routines as the other people in the household, especially if we're the person who holds the traditional role of caregiver. It's amazingly easy for this to happen, considering the number of times in a week, a month, or a year that we prepare food for our families. It all starts with wanting to make sure that we give our family meals which taste good and are satisfying. So, while supper is on the stove, we give it a taste test—a spoonful just to make sure, then we season it a bit more and re-taste it to see if it's better. But, we don't count the food that's already gone into our mouth when we sit down at the table! Those are "hidden" calories that we consume every day, and we don't even think about them.

But wait, there's more. How many times do we go to the grocery store, determined that this time, we'll only buy what we need and everything in the cart will be healthy food that's good for us? Now, try that with a couple of kids by your side. It's as hard as losing weight! Children have a tendency to notice every new cereal, snack bar, and goodie in the store, and the stores are well aware of it, making sure that anything they miss along the way is on display at the checkout, where they're certain to be seen. A short trip for milk, bread, and lettuce can turn into a dieter's nightmare.

If you're serious about changing your eating habits and tightening up your belt a couple of notches, you can't do it without your family. And you shouldn't have to, either. They helped get you where you're at, now, you need them to help you take it off. Tell your family what you're doing and why. Let them know that you want to be healthier for their sake, as well as your own, and that you're asking for their help. Small children love to help, and the older ones will understand if you let them know how important this is to you.

Most importantly, explain to your family that if you're going to be successful, it's going to require a change in the entire family's eating habits. You don't have to restrict all snacks and make everyone miserable, but let them know that from now on, there will be a different variety of snacks available. The regular sweet treats will be occasional, but not standard fare in the house. While they may not be thrilled about it, they will get used to the idea eventually. Like me, you might be surprised to find that your children are just as happy with a snack of granola bites as they were with chocolate chip cookies.

Above all, if at all possible, try to prepare the same meal for your family that you fix for yourself. If you have two meals to cook and choose from, it will be more than a little difficult to lose weight. However, if you learn to prepare healthy food in a healthy way, not only will you lose weight, but your family will also be on their way to a healthier diet and lifestyle. You'll be doing them a favor! Sure, this is your diet, but your health is a family affair.

Chapter Nine

REDECORATE YOUR KITCHEN

When you're trying to lose weight, it's a great time to take a good look at your surroundings. When I did, I found that our kitchen, the heart of our home, was long overdue for a major makeover.

No, I didn't pull out a can of paint or purchase new cabinets. I didn't have to invest in new curtains or flooring. I focused on something entirely different—the food stocked in it.

Staying true and focused while dieting can be challenging, but it's even more so when you have obstacles in your kitchen like potato chips, cookies, and candy. I knew that if I was going to stick to this diet, I was going to have to do some housecleaning and the kitchen was where I had to start.

First, I had a talk with my family, telling them how unhealthy many of our usual staples really are. Sugar coated cereals, cheese puffs, chips, cookies, and snack cakes had to go! From now on, our kitchen is a "heart healthy kitchen."

First, we got rid of everything that was fattening, sugar laden, high calorie, or empty foods. By empty foods, I mean foods which have little or no nutritional value. Then, we replaced them with snacks and foods which are healthy and natural. For instance, out with the Twinkies and in with the Weight Watchers snack cakes. Surprisingly, we found a wide variety of snacks to substitute which we all enjoy. Whole grains, nuts, high fiber cereals, and whole wheat peanut butter crackers are housed in the kitchen now in place of their previous sugary counterparts.

When we finished with the pantry, we turned to the fridge. We now choose skim milk over regular or two percent, and you can usually find several different flavors of yogurt on the shelf. Add to that easy to grab and eat string cheese, fruit, sugar-free pudding, popsicles, etc., and there's something to satisfy everyone in the house!

You might think that eliminating standard sweets and junk food from your family's diet will be difficult. I was surprised to find just how easy it was. My children suddenly took a real interest in the foods they were eating. They've also become more aware of good nutritious food vs. unhealthy ones.

I look around the kitchen now, and I like what I see. There are more options than ever before, and the kitchen is no longer forbidden territory! My kitchen now reflects the lifestyle I want for me and my family. For the first time, I can honestly say that it is the "heart" of our home, and that makes me feel very good!

Chapter Ten

DIETS ARE REWARDING

Diets are reinforcements that we believe we're worthy of being healthier. They're proof that our self-esteem believes we can look better and feel better.

Think about it. What is the biggest reward you receive when you're dieting? It's watching the number on the bathroom scale go lower and your clothes fitting looser, right? What better incentive can you ask for but one which shows you're making real progress and your diet is doing exactly what it's supposed to do?

Yes, progress and weight loss are very rewarding, but there are times when every dieter knows that they need something more. They need a new incentive, something which they can get truly excited about and which will bring them instant gratification along the road toward their long-term goal. That's when rewarding yourself can be just the ticket you need to get past the next hump, meet the next goal, and motivate yourself to keep on keeping on.

Sometimes, it's easier to reach several smaller goals than one big goal. For instance, if you have 20 pounds to lose, you might prefer to set four goals of five pounds each. Then when you reach one goal, you are rewarded with a sense of accomplishment which will keep you motivated to meet the next.

There is something else you can do to inspire yourself to stay on track with your fitness or weight loss goals, and that's to give yourself a special treat when you meet a goal. When you drop your first dress or pant size, buy yourself a new article of clothing to fit the trimmer, more slender body you just created! What a great way to entice yourself to stick with your diet!

You can reward yourself at set increments or when you reach specific milestones. Your personal rewards can be as little or as big as you want them to be. For example, you might treat yourself to a favorite sweet treat after you lose ten pounds, or your incentive might be a promise to yourself that you'll buy a piece of jewelry you've been longing for. Some people might choose to buy a new CD or take a short trip. Others might give themselves a gift of a new exercise video or a new book. Still others might change their hairstyle to match their new look or reward themselves with tickets to a sports game or a play.

No reward is too big or too small. The only thing that matters is that your reward is something you want enough that you'll work towards it. It has to be attractive enough to keep you focused on the goal which is connected to it.

When you do reach your goal and it's time for that long-awaited reward, make sure you acknowledge it. Pat yourself on the back, say Good Job! Give yourself a jump for joy! Feel free to be excited about what you've accomplished and make a celebration out of it. Then, when you give yourself your reward, tell yourself why, congratulating yourself because your hard work and efforts are paying off.

You'll have the body and your own personal reward to prove it!

Chapter Eleven

IT'S A PLAN!

Not only have I found a weight loss program that really works, but I've found a way to increase its chances of success. When I've tried to lose weight in the past, one of the obstacles I faced was a lack of planning. A diet isn't a 24 hour gig—it takes some time to achieve your goals. You have to develop a plan which will get you there.

In the next section of this book, I'm going to share the weight loss plan I've gotten terrific results with, but right now, I want to talk about the importance of planning your day and preparing for any unexpected curves which might get thrown your way.

We've all been caught in the "There's nothing good to eat" situation. Opening the refrigerator, nothing looks appealing. Then, you open the pantry, and nothing looks good there, either. So, you reach for the first thing you can find that's easy to grab and munch on. Wrong! Don't do it! One of the biggest reasons we gain weight in the first place is because we fail to plan our daily meals, and that includes snacks. Designate a specific day each week to plan your weekly menu from morning to night. My day of the week is Saturday. Include breakfast, lunch, dinner, and each and every snack you're going to allow yourself throughout the week. Write it down. Post a seven-day menu on your refrigerator or bulletin board, until the new lifestyle becomes etched in your brain, so you never have to wonder what you are going to eat or if you have the ingredients for that meal.

In that menu, it's important that you also choose a variety of snacks which will tide you over from meal to meal. Be very specific when you plan your snacks and leave no room for substitutions. When I return from the grocery store, where I've bought every item I need for every meal and snack for the entire week, I immediately pre-measure my snacks and place them in containers or zip lock bags, making them convenient to grab and go. This also prevents me from overindulging when I snack. As soon as the contents of that container are gone, I know that I've had my quota and don't reach for more!

Without conscious planning, it's far too easy to reach for foods with a high-calorie content or to eat something which isn't good for our diet simply because we don't have healthy foods available. I've grown dependant on my plan, knowing that it saves me time because I always have everything I need. It also relieves the stress and energy I might otherwise spend debating over what to eat, searching for ingredients, and making trips back and forth to the store (which is never a good idea!). Limiting the number of trips to the grocery store prevents impulse buying, which people often do when they're hungry. Remember, never go to the grocery store on an empty stomach or without your grocery list. It saves on the pocketbook and the hips!

A plan is never complete, though, until it addresses unexpected situations, gatherings, and offerings. Yes, so often we find ourselves in a situation where we're away from home and invited to snack or dine at a meeting, function, or party. Even a short visit to a relative's house will bring invitations to have a cookie, slice of pie, or a drink of your choice. Your plan should always provide you with options for those occasions.

If I'm going to attend a dinner at a restaurant or someone else's home, I make sure I eat a healthy snack before I go. Then, if the menu doesn't include food which is good for my diet, I can either decline it or choose to eat a very small portion without getting too hungry (which is one of the reasons we binge). By preparing before I leave the house, I'm able to make sure that I stick with my plan, and thus, adhere to my new permanent lifestyle.

I like to be able to grab a pre-packaged snack and tuck it in my purse or pocket before I leave the house, just in case I'm gone for a longer period of time than I anticipate. Therefore, I don't find myself in a position where I have to resort to fast food or eating something which isn't good for me. Society gives us far too many reasons to cheat, so I've found that I have to carry healthy options with me at all times.

While it may sound like some work planning a menu and prepackaging your snacks, it's actually a lot less work and trouble than winging it. Once you do it for a couple of weeks, it will become so routine that you'll wonder why no one ever recommended this to you years ago. You don't have to fret over your diet and what you're going to eat, shop and spend more money than absolutely necessary, and you're free all week long from decision making, measuring, or wondering if what you're eating is good for you. After the first week or two, you begin to look forward to writing your weekly plan. It makes you feel confident, organized and in control, keeps you on track, and helps you resist a dieter's worst enemy— temptation!

Chapter Twelve

LAST, BUT NOT LEAST

Before we delve into your weight-loss plan, I want to take a moment to address an issue that many people struggle with in losing weight—eating. Far too many people think of a diet as a food deprivation plan, meaning that we reduce the amount of food we eat. That could be one reason why so many people have difficulty staying on a diet. They don't allow themselves enough food to satisfy their hunger or to nourish their body.

I'd like you to change your attitude about weight loss. A diet doesn't forbid eating, and it doesn't mean that you have to starve. It simply means that you have to alter the foods you do eat and be more sensible about what you choose to nourish your body and how much of it you consume.

Take an honest look at the foods you eat. Are you getting sustenance when you eat, or are you getting empty calories which have little or no nutritional value? If you choose sensibly, you'll be able to eat healthy foods which taste good and bc able to eat enough of them to satisfy your hunger pangs until your next snack or meal. Real hunger should never be part of your weight loss plan!

So, change your mindset when you change your eating habits. Look at it this way: A diet is about the foods you eat—not the foods you don't eat. Don't think of a diet as a plan to deprive yourself—think of it as a plan to nourish yourself. Stop thinking of it as a starving program—start thinking of it as an eating program. After all, hunger is a dieter's recipe for failure. Feed your hunger and feed your body.

Redefine the word diet so it gives you permission to eat and enjoy food. Food is fuel for the body. Giving your body what it needs will satisfy your cravings, curb your hunger, and keep you on track toward your goal. There are so many options to help you do that—weigh them and choose the ones which will create your own success story!

SECTION TWO:

THE DIET

Chapter Thirteen

WEIGHING THE OPTIONS

So, you've made a conscious decision to lose weight. That's great, but it's not enough. Wanting to lose weight is the first step to making it happen, but it's going to take more than that. If only it were that easy!

While dieting is never extremely easy, we do hear and read about diets which are supposedly painless. There are pills which claim to melt away fat and suppress our ravishing appetites. There are other pills which are supposed to increase our metabolism so we burn more fat. There are many different weight-loss programs, as well. Most of these require that you purchase a specific type of food and/or pay a membership fee. The bad part is, while they do work for a while, most people regain the weight they lose on these plans as soon as they go off their diet.

I won't claim that dieting is easy, but it doesn't have to be that hard, either. It doesn't always have to result in regaining the pounds lost when we resume our normal eating habits. Diets don't have to deprive us of sweet treats or carbohydrates. They don't have to overdose our bodies on grapefruits and cottage cheese, either. The best diet in the world is the one that works for you, your eating habits, and your lifestyle. Also, the best diet in the world doesn't have to cost an arm and a leg. As a matter of fact, eating right is probably less expensive than indulging in sweets, junk food, and foods which are high in fat or sugars.

The best diet in the world actually has three main ingredients—that's Protein, Fiber and Perseverance! Will power is often the missing ingredient in diets, which is one reason why so many fail. But, I've found a way to lose weight that doesn't test my will power every time I turn around because it allows me to eat the foods I love and that keep me satisfied between meals. It gives me the freedom to choose what I want to eat, when I want to eat it, and removes the guesswork out of the equation.

When I came to the conclusion that I needed to do something about my weight, I did some research. Anyone can get on the Internet and find millions of different weight-loss solutions. Walk into a bookstore and you'll find a wide variety of books claiming to have the answer to your overweight woes. But I was looking for something more. I wanted to find a diet which would produce consistent, visible results, but which was also convenient and easy to follow. I also wanted a diet that wasn't too drastic, but which would help me maintain the weight once I took it off. Was I asking too much? I didn't think so.

Then, it dawned on me. The answer to losing weight wasn't in a pill, a fad, or a gimmick. It didn't mean I had to join a program or an exercise club. I didn't have to starve myself or eat raw vegetables non-stop for the next two months. Losing weight wasn't rocket science—it was common sense.

I'd gained weight because of one thing—I ate more than my body needed and had been on one diet after another for years and had messed up my metabolism by doing so. If I changed that, my weight woes would be history. I had to figure out just how much food my body needed. How much was I overeating, and how much did I have to cut back?

To find the answer, I logged onto the Internet and did a search…I wanted to know how much I should actually weigh, given my age, height and body structure. Then, I'd know just how much weight I had to lose. I found many weight tables with varying ranges, but after looking at two or three, I had a good idea of how much extra baggage I was carrying. I also found that there is no "ideal" weight for a specific person, just an "ideal" weight range. That was good—it gave me a little wiggle room and the ability to choose a weight which was healthy and comfortable for me.

There is one easy way to gauge your ideal weight, and it brings you very close to the ideal or desired weight in the weight tables I found. Here's the equation:

WOMEN:

Five feet tall: 100 pounds

Add an additional 5 pounds for every inch over 5 feet.

MEN:

Five feet tall: 106 pounds

Add an additional 6 pounds for every inch over 5 feet.

Now, compare that weight to the desired weight ranges in the following tables:

WOMEN

(Determine your frame by wrapping your thumb and index finger around your wrist. If they overlap, you have a small frame. If they meet, you have a medium frame. If they don't meet, use the column for large frame to determine your desired weight range.)

HEIGHT	SMALL FRAME	MEDIUM FRAME	LARGE FRAME
4'10"	102-111	109-121	118-131
4'11"	103-113	111-123	120-134
5'0"	104-115	113-126	122-137
5'1"	106-118	115-129	125-140
5'2"	108-121	118-132	128-143
5'3"	111-124	121-135	131-147
5'4"	114-127	124-138	134-151
5'5"	117-130	127-141	137-155
5'6"	120-133	130-144	140-159
5'7"	123-136	133-147	143-163
5'8"	126-139	136-150	146-167
5'9"	129-142	139-153	149-170
5'10"	132-145	142-156	152-173
5'11"	135-148	145-159	155-176
6'0"	138-151	148-162	158-179

*Ideal Weights according to the Metropolitan Life Insurance Company tables (1983)

MEN			
(Determine your frame by wrapping your thumb and index finger around your wrist. If they overlap, you have a small frame. If they meet, you have a medium frame. If they don't meet, use the column for large frame to determine your desired weight range.)			
EIGHT	**SMALL FRAME**	**MEDIUM FRAME**	**LARGE FRAME**
5'2"	128-134	131-141	138-150
5'3"	130-136	133-143	140-153
5'4"	132-138	135-145	142-156
5'5"	134-140	137-148	144-160
5'6"	136-142	139-151	146-164
5'7"	138-145	142-154	149-168
5'8"	140-148	145-157	152-172
5'9"	142-151	148-160	155-176
5'10"	144-154	151-163	158-180
5'11"	146-157	154-166	161-184
6'0"	149-160	157-170	164-188
6'1"	152-164	160-174	168-192
6'2"	155-168	164-178	172-197
6'3"	158-172	167-182	176-202
6'4"	162-176	171-187	181-207

*Ideal Weights according to the Metropolitan Life Insurance Company tables (1983)

As you can see, there's more "wiggle room" in the weight ranges listed in these charts than there probably is in your favorite pair of jeans. Only you know the weight where you feel most comfortable, healthy, and which is easiest for you to maintain.

I know that height/weight charts and ideal weights aren't anything new. This chart was made in 1983, and there certainly might be revisions in the future. However, they are a good gauge of the medical standards for a healthy body weight.

Once I determined how much I should weigh, I knew my work was cut out for me. The pounds didn't creep up overnight, and I was aware that they wouldn't melt away that fast, either. However, I wanted a weight-loss plan that would work as quickly as possible! So, here's what I did to lose 15 pounds in one month, so I'm a testament to its success. I figured out how many calories I could eat to maintain my "DESIRED" weight—not to maintain my current weight, but my desired weight. That number became the amount of calories which I would consume over the course of a day in order to lose weight. What I found was that I could lose weight on a steady basis by adjusting my food intake or increasing my activity.

We've all heard of the 1,000 or 1,200 calorie a day diet, which is torture! It's too hard to follow those diets; they simply don't provide enough calories a day to curb hunger. One sure way to make sure you don't stick to a diet is to starve! The secret to dieting isn't finding a 1,200 calorie diet—it's eating as many calories as your body will need at its ideal or desired weight. Lo and behold, that answer also provided me with the knowledge I needed to maintain that weight once I got there!

Curbing my calories was the option I chose to lose weight. Finding the daily calorie count for the weight I wanted to be was a little more difficult, but I did come across a really neat calorie counter on the American Cancer Society's website (visit it at: http://www.cancer.org/docroot/PED/content/PED_6_1x_Calorie_Calculator.asp).

All I had to do was input my weight (or in this case, the weight I wanted to be) to find out how many calories I could eat and stay at that weight! The site takes into consideration your lifestyle and how active you are, and I chose a sedentary lifestyle.

If you want to take the guesswork (and room for error) out of your weight-loss plan, I suggest that you also choose a sedentary or limited activity lifestyle. When you do, you'll know that the calorie count suggested will actually be right. If you are moderately active, that's okay, because you'll lose more weight at a faster pace by choosing a sedentary activity level.

While that's not all there is to losing weight, it's a very good start! Knowing how much you want to weigh and how many calories you should intake to get there and maintain that weight is half of the battle!

Just how fast will the weight come off? That depends on you, your metabolism, your activity level, and how closely you follow your diet. Realistically, there is no way to lose a massive amount of weight overnight (short of liposuction); after all, arriving at a plus size happened one potato chip, cookie, and extra helping at a time. It came about by snacking and because I got a tad bit lazy in not being conscious and paying attention to everything I did eat. Not to mention, I didn't have the tools or knowledge to go along with all of the above. I'd forgotten much of what I learned in school about food and nutrition and lost sight of the fact that there are 3,500 calories in a pound. However, I never lost sight of the pounds packed on by the extra calories I consumed! It doesn't seem like much, but over time, one extra cookie a day can add inches to the waist line.

The great news is that the reverse is also true—deduct 3,500 calories and you'll lose a pound! Now, we all know that it's not realistic and is dangerous to deprive our body of food, so we don't want to drastically reduce our caloric intake. We simply have to modify it so it fits the person we want to be, not the person we've become. There is no need for starvation, deprivation, or strenuous physical exercise. The plan works all by itself. The sheer beauty of it is in its simplicity. Are you ready for a slimmer, trimmer you? Do you want to feel good, look good, and know precisely what it will take to stay that way? Then, please join me as I share my diet tips and tricks with you and show you that losing weight is actually easier than you ever thought possible.

Chapter Fourteen

PLANNING YOUR DIET

Once I got past the point of planning to diet, I had to plan my diet. I already knew exactly how much I wanted to weigh and how many calories I could eat a day to get there. I'd seen my physician and had heeded his advice. Now, I had to figure out what I could (and couldn't) eat.

To plan my daily diet, I took the total calories allowed for the day and divided them between breakfast, lunch, supper, and two snacks. You can divide your calories however you wish, which is the beauty of this diet plan. Some people like to eat a heavier breakfast, while others prefer a lighter meal in the morning and a more substantial one later in the day. Regardless, I make sure there is room in my daily menu for two snacks every day. Giving myself a 100 or 150 calorie snack in the morning and in the afternoon tides me over until the next meal and keeps me from feeling deprived. I know what I can eat and how many calories it contains, so by snacking, I'm not cheating. Because I plan my snacks, I'm preventing myself from falling privy to eating without being aware of it!

The one thing I love about this diet is the freedom it gives me. I can choose the foods I like and eat them when I feel like it, as long as I don't exceed my daily calorie count. The problem I've found in the past was that I wasn't paying attention to everything that went in my mouth. That's why I became just a little shocked when I realized how much weight I'd gained. This is a common theme among women and men who gain weight—they don't "count" everything that goes in their mouth, but their hips aren't quite as forgiving!

A little bit here and a little bit there might apply to eating, but it also applies to excess weight. Tasting food as we cook counts. So, too, does grabbing a cracker, a cookie, three or four M & M's, or a handful of chips. We don't even count that as eating, but it is. So, what's a girl to do? Be honest, totally and brutally honest, and write down each and every little morsel you eat. If you're like me, you'll be surprised at how many hidden calories there are in your daily diet.

Begin today to keep a journal, where you write down what you eat, how much of it you ate, and the calories it contained. Include everything, even drinks, which we often neglect to consider. One can of regular soda packs about 150 calories—one or two of those a day is enough to make you gain weight, instead of losing it!

The purpose of your journal at first is to make you aware of how often you eat. For many of us, it's the unconscious eating (when we're standing, driving, watching TV, etc.) that caused us to gain weight. Your journal will create awareness of what you eat, and before long, you'll think before you reach for a cracker or a cookie, knowing that those little bites and nibbles here and there are contributing to your weight gain.

The biggest tip I can give you is to use your journal to develop full insight of your eating habits. Include not only everything you eat and drink, but also write down why you ate it. Were you hungry? Were you bored? Were you sad or angry? What time of day was it? We all have different reasons for opening the pantry—use your journal to help you find your reasons. When you do, you'll also begin to pay attention to your mood and attitude and know that there are times when you have to run, not walk, away from the kitchen!

Chapter Fifteen

WRAP IT UP

This weight loss plan really does work, but only if you count every calorie that goes into your mouth. There's an old saying that the food we eat goes straight to our hips. While that's not entirely true, it can seem that way, especially if we don't know why we're gaining weight in the first place. One of the biggest reasons I found that I had gained weight over time is because I wasn't aware of just how many calories I consumed on a daily basis.

Once I started paying attention to the calorie content of the foods I eat, I've become a huge fan of nutrition labels. Prepackaged foods contain nutrition labels which tell us exactly how much food is in a single serving size and how many calories it contains. It takes all the work out of the journal and makes planning a daily and weekly meal plan effortless!

Prepackaged foods offer a great deal of convenience. Taking advantage of individually wrapped servings can save a lot of time and effort. In addition, there has never been a wider variety of prepackaged snacks available to the consumer.

I'm a fan of prepackaged meals and entrees for meals. There has never been a wider variety of foods geared toward health consciousness and weight loss than there is today. Many manufacturers market prepared meals which contain healthy ingredients in individual proportions which are tasty enough to eat, even when you're not dieting! One look in your grocer's freezer, and you'll be sure to find a wide assortment of Lean Cuisine, Weight Watchers, Healthy Choice, and other entrees from which to select. In addition, they include many of our favorite foods, including pizza, lasagna, chicken, or beef stew (just to name a very few!)

How much easier can it get! These foods are already prepared, you simply have to heat and eat, and they've already done the calorie counting for you. You know precisely what you're eating and how many of your daily calories you're using with each and every dish. There's no risk of overserving yourself or temptation to have a second helping. The added bonus is that you don't have messy bowls, pots or pans to clean up when you're done!

I also depend on prepackaged food for my snacks. Many companies have jumped on the bandwagon and now provide individually wrapped servings. Some of these are specifically marketed based on their calorie count, and for those which aren't, one glance at the nutrition label on the box or package will tell you precisely how many calories there are in an individual serving size. For instance, granola bars, mini muffins, crackers, and even cookies come in individually wrapped serving sizes which contain precisely 100 calories. That's perfect fare for a morning or afternoon snack. Depending on how many calories you allot toward each snack, you can grab one or two and know exactly how many calories you're intaking.

Other prepackaged food options include string cheese, yogurt, canned soup, individual serving sizes of tuna, chicken, pasta, vegetables, and potato or rice dishes. It makes it easy to have something different every day, while ensuring that I don't exceed my daily quota of calories. Eating a wide variety of foods, spices, flavors and textures is important to a diet because it helps keep boredom at bay, which is often when dieters cheat. Besides that, many of the prepackaged foods available are flavorful and tasty enough that it doesn't seem like I'm dieting at all!

Some foods, however, aren't individually wrapped in proportioned serving sizes. That's when you need to read and understand the nutrition label so you can ensure that you're not exceeding your caloric limit. Nutrition labels also provide valuable information about fat, sugar, fiber, vitamin and mineral content for those who are health conscious. The last section of this book contains information on how to read nutrition labels so you can take full advantage of the information contained in them.

When I do choose a snack that isn't already prepackaged and wrapped for me, I measure and wrap snack size portions myself. After doing my weekly shopping, I take a few minutes to make my snack bags, putting individual servings in containers or zip lock bags that are easy to grab and go.

For instance, if I allow myself to have a 125 calorie snack in the morning and another in the afternoon, I measure and package the right amount of food to meet that requirement and don't have to think about it again. I can grab one or two before I leave the house in the morning and reach for them when I'm away from home, driving, or when I'm tempted to take a trip to the vending machine.

The upside of prepackaged foods is that many brands make entrees which would be a lot of work to cook at home. They introduce different tastes and spices to what could be a boring diet, so much so, that even people who aren't dieting like them! The trick to finding what works for you is to stick with food that you're familiar with or which fits into your normal diet. For instance, if you like to have Mexican food once a week, you'll probably be quite content with one of the prepackaged brands of burritos or quesadillas. You can also cheat a little without cheating by choosing some of the sweet treats and desserts available. Frozen and prepackaged foods don't have to taste like cardboard! After all, dieting doesn't mean you can't enjoy food. Like little Mikey, in the Life cereal commercial, you might be pleasantly surprised and find that you do like it after all!

Chapter Sixteen

SPEED IT UP

It seems like common sense that if you're trying to lose weight, you should reduce how much you eat and how often you eat, right? Wrong!

Our body has this thing called metabolism, which works almost without fail. There are some dieters who immediately cut back on meals and go into near starvation mode in order to lose weight, but it won't cause them to lose a drastic amount of weight in a short period of time because of one thing: metabolism.

Metabolism is how your body converts calories to energy. It has a basic purpose: survival.

Here's how it works. When you eat food, your body uses X number of calories for energy. Consume more calories than your body needs, and the excess calories are stored as fat for future energy use. It's kind of like stocking up at the grocery store. You might buy more than you need, but you store it for later use. Well, your body does the same thing, and says, "Whoa, there's more calories here than I need today, so I'm just going to store them until later when I need them." Thus, fat is born.

So, your body is protecting you and making sure that you have enough energy to survive later.

But, when you diet and reduce your calories, metabolism doesn't work in quite the same way. Reducing the amount of food you eat and how often you eat actually slows your metabolism down, causing your body to burn fewer calories.

In the following scenario, think of calories as energy, where the food we eat produces the energy our body needs. Dee goes on a diet, reasoning that the less food she eats, the faster she'll lose weight. Dan, another dieter, also starts a weight loss program, but he makes sure that he eats. His plan involves changing the foods he eats, while ensuring he eats three meals and a couple snacks a day. Who will lose weight faster?

To answer that question, let's see how Dee's body responds to her minimal eating plan. Dee's body uses the calories it needs for the day, but also notices that there aren't any more calories coming in to address her daily energy needs. So, her body does precisely what it's intended to do and goes into survival mode. First, her metabolism slows down, making sure that she burns fewer calories to compensate for the lack of calories coming in. Her metabolism stops burning the calories she does consume and starts saving (or storing) them for later use. It's kind of like rationing. If we hear there's going to be a shortage of gasoline, we could fill gas cans and save them so we have plenty when the supply is tight. Dee's body is doing the same with energy, making sure that she'll have stored energy during her period of deprivation. In addition, her body's energy supply is now drastically reduced, so it must find a source of energy for her current needs. That energy usually comes from the protein in the muscle. You see, the body is well aware that protein is a better source of energy than fat! So, while her body uses her muscles to survive, the stored fat sits right where it's at and won't be touched until the protein sources are tapped. Meanwhile, her current efforts to lose weight aren't very effective because her metabolism has slowed down drastically.

Dan, on the other hand, is reducing the number of calories he's eating, but ensuring he gets enough to provide him with the necessary energy he needs. He's eating foods high in protein, but lower in calories. He's eating three healthy, balanced meals each day and supplementing them with two healthy snacks between meals. Dan is losing weight by eating than Dee is by starving. Why? First, because Dan is eating and giving his body the nutrition and energy it needs, his metabolism doesn't have to slow down. In fact, it's speeding up. Dan's metabolism rate increases to burn the calories he's consuming, unlike Dee, who's metabolism slows down to compensate for the lack of calories she consumes. Because Dan is eating, he's losing more weight than Dee, who is eating very little.

We've all known someone who claims that they don't eat, but they just can't seem to lose weight. They are a victim of their metabolism. It's probably very true that they don't eat often, and their body responded just like it's supposed to—it went into survival mode, slowing down their metabolism and storing calories during what the body perceives to be a crisis. What they don't know is that if they really want to lose weight, they have to do the one thing they're not doing---EAT!

There are some things you can do to speed up your metabolism even further, and that's one of the keys to losing more weight at a faster pace. Here are a few suggestions:

- Eat three meals a day. The issue is what you eat—not whether you eat.

- Breakfast is the most important meal of the day. Your body has been deprived of new energy since you went to bed the night before, so your metabolism is already slowing down. Eat a healthy breakfast and kick start it back into high gear.

- Eat snacks. Snacks will keep your metabolism functioning at an even level, preventing your body's signals for more energy. Remember, though, to keep your snacks healthy and don't exceed the calorie count you allow for snacks.

- There are certain times of the day when your body really does need more energy and calories than others. Eat larger meals and snacks during the times when you are most active and busy to make sure you have a sufficient amount of energy to keep your metabolism at a higher level.

- Make sure you drink plenty of water to stay hydrated. The extra benefit is that water helps metabolism to perform at its best.

- Exercise regularly. When you exercise, your metabolic rate speeds up and it doesn't return to normal for a couple hours after you're done exercising!

So, if you're like me and you really do want to lose weight and do it as quickly as possible, you must eat. Eat foods which are good for you and high in protein. Eat when you're active. Eat in the morning. Eat between meals. Eating is not a dieter's enemy, but eating the right foods at the right times can be a dieter's very best friend.

Chapter Seventeen

CHEATER, CHEATER

Why do diets fail? Diets fail because people cave into temptation and they cheat! Once they cheat, they figure they might as well keep eating because they've wrecked their diet...for today, anyway.

The beauty of this diet is that you can cheat if and when you want to! If you have a sweet tooth, you can indulge in an occasional cookie or bowl of ice cream without undoing everything you've accomplished. You can give yourself permission to cheat. You simply have to fit it into your daily (or weekly) calorie count.

There are times when we get hungry for some of our favorite foods. There will be occasions, like birthdays, anniversaries, or special dinners, when we are expected to or want to eat something that we know will wreak havoc on our diet. Does that mean that we can't occasionally 'cheat' just a little and have a slice of birthday cake or enjoy the prime rib dinner at the annual company party? No, it doesn't. If that happens, you simply have to adjust your eating plan for that day or the week.

You can do that in several different ways. Neither is right or wrong—it depends on what works for you, your routine, and your schedule.

One way to cheat without cheating is to pre-plan. If you know that you'll be attending a birthday party that day, you can cut back on the calories in that day's meals or substitute a small slice of cake for your two snacks. You can substitute fruits and veggies for a higher calorie lunch, if you wish. That's why this diet is easy to follow. You know your limits, but you also have total freedom over the foods you choose to reach your quota.

The other way you can cheat without tossing your whole diet to the wind, which works really well if you don't have an opportunity to preplan. Sometimes, impromptu food offerings are too irresistible to pass up. In that case, go ahead, splurge a little (don't overdo it!) Just make sure you remember to write it down! Then, get back on track for the rest of the day or the rest of the week by trimming back the calories you consume during those days to accommodate the treat you've given yourself.

The last way you can cheat without feeling guilty about it is to preplan for the entire week. If you know that there's something you really want, say a slice of pecan pie, then determine how many calories are in that slice of pie and curb a few calories off your intake everyday. Then, when Saturday comes and it's time to enjoy your craving, you'll have enough unused calories to indulge! It's like rolling calories over at the end of the day for future use!

I really think that it's important to occasionally eat foods which I enjoy, but which I know aren't in my daily diet plan. When I do, it satisfies my cravings and gives me permission to enjoy a temptation without crashing my diet. Feeling deprived is a huge morale breaker, and it's one of the biggest reasons people can't stick to a diet plan for the duration. Knowing that I can accommodate a treat by pre or post-planning keeps me on track toward my goal. As a bonus, it provides me with an incentive to stay true to my new lifestyle for the rest of the day or week!

SECTION THREE:

TOOLS AND RESOURCES YOU CAN USE

Chapter Eighteen

NEED HELP? GET A COACH

People have turned to coaches to meet sales goals, as well as other professional and personal goals. A coach is someone who applies their expertise and experience to another person's particular situation, and advises, motivates, and challenges them to meet specific goals and improve areas where they are weak. Dieting comes with challenges. It's not something we can accomplish overnight. It takes perseverance, will power, commitment and patience. Sometimes, we need support. There will be times when we need someone who will be objective and honest, telling us what we're doing right and what we're doing wrong. That's why I recommend that people who are serious about losing weight and living a healthier lifestyle seek the services of a weight loss coach.

I used to have a weight loss coach, and she offered me so many good suggestions that I use. The coach's job is not to devise your diet plan, but to provide you with the encouragement and tools to follow the plan you have. They want you to succeed and are trained to identify your weaknesses and show you ways to strengthen them and to overcome the obstacles and challenges you'll face along the way.

For instance, a weight loss coach can work with you to identify the emotional triggers which create a desire to eat, like boredom, loneliness, stress, or worry. He or she will have a stock of good suggestions you can apply to become aware of and control any bouts of unconscious eating (those times when you reach for snacks like cookies or chips and eat without being truly aware of what or how much you're really consuming).

A weight loss coach is trained to help you identify what works for you. They know that no two people are alike and that we all have different reasons and circumstances which contributed to our weight gain. They'll partner with you to find a plan that works for you and to set realistic, measurable goals to work toward. Your own personal weight loss coach can help you break bad habits and replace them with a foundation of healthier ones which you can use during and after your diet.

Above all, a weight loss coach provides us with the motivation that too often wanes as our diet goes on. Reminding us of our emotional and physical desire to be thin and the benefits which we'll derive from dropping excess pounds, they keep us on track and self disciplined as we focus on our goal.

If you think you're in this alone, I strongly encourage you to find a weight loss, diet or fitness coach. At the end of this Book are several links and references to weight loss coaches and motivating articles with tips and tricks to keep you on track. Use them as a resource to better health or find your own personal weight loss coach to guide and motivate you. They want you to succeed and will help you to believe that failure is not a possibility!

Chapter Nineteen

JOURNAL YOUR JOURNEY

One of the great things about this diet plan is that it works. Unlike other diets, there are no special foods which you must eat or foods which you absolutely have to avoid. You have options and total control over what you eat and when you eat! In essence, this diet provides freedom which many other diets restrict.

However, this diet will only work if you're totally honest with yourself. You must acknowledge every morsel, bite, and snack that goes into your mouth. Neglecting to count calories is a recipe for failure! That's why I promote, encourage and use a journal, documenting the food I eat every day, every last bite. To make it as easy and painless as possible, I'm providing you with a sample of a simple journal you can use to log your daily food intake. There are several good ones online which you can also access at no cost or you can make your own on the computer or on a plain sheet of paper. I like to use the journal online or put it in an electronic spreadsheet because it automatically adds my total calorie intake every day.

I've taken the liberty of filling out a sample daily log because I want to show you how I complete my journal and give you an idea of just how calorie rich some foods are! Being aware that foods which are extremely high in calories will rob you of an opportunity to enjoy your other meals throughout the day will help you to steer clear of them, so you can enjoy faster results.

DAILY FOOD LOG

DATE			
FOOD	**QUANTITY**	**CALORIES**	**MOOD**

Below is an example of a food log or journal which has been completed.

Date	Time	Food	Amount/Quantity	Mood / Activity	Calories
Jan. 1	7 am	Coffee with 1 tsp. sugar Frosted Flakes and milk	1 cup ¾ cup ½ cup	Tired, getting kids ready for school	15 110 40
	10 am	Granola bar	1	Stressed, returning emails	100
	11:15	Potato chips	15	Bored, driving	150
	12:30	Fast food cheeseburger French fries soda pop	1 Small Medium	Rushed, running errands	310 210 210
					1,250

As you can see by the chart, by lunch time, you've consumed 1,250 calories! If your daily calorie intake for your desired weight is 1,500, you've almost met your quota and you have plenty of day and night ahead of you! Keeping track of everything you eat will open your eyes to not only how much you eat, but how often you eat! I purposely included fast food in this example because I wanted you to see just how calorie-rich it is.

At the end of the day, go back and review your log. Is there a certain time of the day when hunger hits or when you get bored? If you know that, you can try to quell those hunger pangs with a more nutritious snack than potato chips. This is also a very good indicator of the times in your daily routine when you need to find something to do. Let's say you're bored between 10:30 and noon. At 10:30, switch gears and do something different! Visit that one thing you're passionate about and spend an hour and a half working on it. You can also try getting up, moving around, finding a change of scenery—anything to divert your time and attention so you don't eat when you're not hungry, which has killed many a diet.

The key to making this journal work for you, not only as a tracking tool, but to keep yourself on track, is to make sure you don't leave a single thing out. Include everything you eat, no matter how small it might be. You have to be totally honest with yourself because ignoring or forgiving 100 calories (like those 15 potato chips) is enough to keep your diet from working, and actually might be the cause of further weight gain!

If you log your daily intake on the computer, make sure you keep a small notebook with you at all times so you don't forget to write anything down. The calorie count from foods can be obtained online, in mini books (like you find in the checkout lane at the grocery store) or from the nutrition labels on packaged foods. I've included several excellent print and online resources in the back of this book which I think you might enjoy. They are an excellent resource you can use to accurately record the calorie content of the foods you eat.

Once you have that information in hand, you can go back and look at places where you can alter your diet. How many calories would you save by choosing a healthier lunch or by packing your own lunch? Do you eat when you're not hungry? Can you substitute a snack which has fewer calories, or would it be enough to simply reduce your serving size?

Everyone's answers will depend on their own eating habits. I found that I eat when I'm bored and shortly after eating a refined sugar meal or snack, often without thinking about it. By finding something else to consume my time and attention rather than my appetite, I was able to cut a large chunk of extra calories out of my diet. I also came to the conclusion that a lot of the foods I was snacking on were empty calories (full of sugar or fat) and I could substitute something which had fewer calories and was more filling. I eat protein and/or fiber at every meal. If I do eat something sweet, it has no more than 16 grams of sugar or less, along with protein or fiber (or a combination of both) so my insulin level stays balanced and my body is able to release the fat from my cells. In many cases, I didn't have to reduce the amount of food I ate at all. I just had to make better choices!

Chapter Twenty

READING NUTRITION LABELS

Throughout this book, I've also supported eating foods which are prepackaged and contain calorie and nutrition information on the package's nutrition label. While certain kinds of food may contain an approximate number of calories, each individual brand may contain either more or less, depending on the ingredients and how the food is made. That's why I depend on nutrition labels to provide me with the most accurate information for the specific foods I eat.

Be careful when reading nutrition labels, though. Pay particular attention to serving size. A food produce that you believe contains one serving size might actually contain two or three! Always refer to the serving size for cereal, some are smaller than others. Contrary to popular belief, the serving size for cereal is not one bowl – but actually ½ to ¾ of a cup! Eating a full bowl of cereal will double or triple your calorie count!

I also use nutrition labels to become educated on other dietary contents in foods I eat. If you have certain health conditions, the information becomes even more important. That's why I've included definitions for the information included in nutrition labels and the role it plays in our diet and overall health.

A standard nutrition label will include the following information:

- Serving Size & Servings Per Container/Package
- Calories per serving

- Calories from Fat per serving
- Total Saturated and Trans Fat
- Sodium
- Carbohydrates, including fiber, sugars, and glycerin
- Protein
- Nutritional Content, such as:
  - Calcium
  - Iron
  - Vitamins
  - Other minerals
  - Percentage of Daily Values

While some of that information may seem somewhat technical, once you know how to read the nutritional labels on packaged food, the process is simplified. Let's start by looking at an example of a nutrition label for a granola bar:

Serving Size	1 bar (24 g)	
Servings Per Container	4	
Calories per Serving	100	
Calories from Fat	30	
		% DV (daily value)
Total Fat	3.5g	6%

Saturated Fat	1g	6%
Trans Fat	0g	
Sodium	75mg	3%
Total Carbohydrate		
Dietary Fiber		
Sugars		
Glycerin		
Protein	1g	
Calcium		10%
Iron		2%

People with health issues, like high cholesterol, heart disease, hypertension, and high or low blood sugar should pay particular attention to the fat, sugar, and sodium levels in the food they eat. Regardless if you're dieting to lose weight or controlling a health condition, you should understand what the specific categories of a food label mean. Let's look at them now.

Fat: Fat is divided into two categories: Saturated Fat and Trans Fat.

- Saturated Fat: Saturated fat is credited with contributing to heart disease, stroke, and high cholesterol levels. There is also some evidence that there may be an association between diets high in saturated fat and breast cancer and prostate cancer. Therefore, it is suggested that whenever possible saturated fat be replaced with polyunsaturated fat. The American Heart Association suggests limiting saturated fat in our diets to less than 7% of our total calorie intake. Therefore, if you're trying to eat healthier, pay close attention to the amount of saturated fat in the foods you eat.

- Trans Fat: Trans Fat plays a significant role in cholesterol levels. It is actually a double edged sword. Trans Fat is charged with lowering good cholesterol, otherwise known as HDL, which is actually good for you because it removes excess cholesterol from the body by sending it to the liver. Trans Fat also raises bad cholesterol, commonly referred to as LDL. LDL cholesterol is the one that builds up in arteries, causing them to narrow and harden. An increase in triglycerides (another type of fat) and inflammation can also result from eating foods high in trans fat. For those reasons, physicians view Trans Fat (or Trans Fatty Acids) as the worst type of fat.

Trans Fat is produced from hydrogenation, a process which adds hydrogen to standard vegetable oil. This process helps prevent spoiling because trans fat is more solid than oil. It's used in the food industry to lengthen the freshness of food and give them a less greasy consistency.

The controversy in trans fats in the fact that it was once considered to be healthier than animal fat because it is derived from plants and is also unsaturated. Over the years, though, there are has been considerable evidence of the damage it does to cholesterol levels.

Being knowledgeable is your best weapon against trans fat. While many manufacturers have taken a proactive approach and limited or eliminated the use of trans fat in the foods they make, there are certain foods which still contain trans fat. Commercially baked goods are one of them. These contain certain cookies, cakes, and crackers. Trans fat is also present in some fried food, like french fries and donuts. In its purest form, it can be found in some margarines and shortening.

Nutrition labels will tell you if trans fat is present, but they can be deceiving. Companies are only required to disclose trans fat at levels of 0.5 grams or higher per serving. That means that they can claim that anything less than that contains 0% trans fat. Eating multiple items with some trans fat, but less than 0.5 grams per serving, can be bad for you. So, a word to the wise is to look at the ingredients in the food you eat. If it includes shortening, there is probably some trans fat in the food. In addition, "partially hydrogenated" vegetable oil is another term for trans fat. Steer clear of any food which contains those words. The same is true if the ingredient is labeled as just "hydrogenated," because it probably also contains trace levels of trans fat. You're okay with fully hydrogenated oils because they don't contain trans fatty acids. Dairy product and meat can also contain trans fats, but they are considered safer—it's the trans fat in processed foods which is deemed to be particularly bad for you.

Society is becoming more conscious of the negative effects of trans fat; however, it is still present in foods and used in oils by some restaurants. The nutrition label you see on foods won't list the percentage daily value for trans fats because it's still not know what an accepted or appropriate level is. The one thing that is known is that the level of trans fat in our diet should be low. Some suggest that trans fat should not exceed more than one percent of our daily caloric intake, meaning that a 1,500 calorie diet should have no more than 1.5 grams of trans fat per day.

Trans fats can be replaced by using plant oils, but you should know that those contain saturated fats. While saturated fats are the lesser of the two evils, they still raise your bad cholesterol level. To maintain a healthy diet and a healthy heart, no more than 30 percent of your daily calories should come from fat. Better yet, choose monounsaturated fat, which you'll find in peanut, canola, and olive oil.

Sodium: The diet of the average adult contains 4,000 to 6,000 mg of Sodium. However, it is suggested that we should limit our sodium intake to 2,400 mg. People on sodium restricted diets should further reduce that amount to a level recommended by their physician or dietician. Sodium is used to flavor food (think of salt), to preserve food (think again of salt), and to stabilize food. One teaspoon of salt contains about 2,000 mg of sodium, almost an entire day's recommended allotment.

Sodium is required to be included on nutrition labels because it is a factor in controlling hypertension (high blood pressure). Reducing the amount of sodium in your diet will reduce your blood pressure, also reducing your risk of heart disease. Sodium is typically introduced into our diet through the use of salt. This includes more than the salt we add to the food we make and eat—it also includes salt in processed foods, like canned goods, frozen food, and packaged convenience foods, which include high levels of preservatives. Some levels of sodium are naturally present in the foods and beverages we eat and drink, like some meats, fish, milk and cheese. In addition, hidden sources of sodium are contained in chicken, lamb, and kosher beef because salt is added to those before they are packaged to delay the spoiling process.

Sugars: While sugars are included on nutrition labels, the label won't include a daily percent value because there is not an established recommended percentage of sugar intake. The sugars which are included on labels include natural sugars, which are present in fruit and milk, and also sugars which are added to food and beverages. Corn syrup, granulated and brown sugar, honey, syrup, sucrose, maltose, dextrose, and fruit juice concentrate are common forms of added sugars. Each of these sugars has a different calorie count. It's recommended that no more than 15 percent of your daily calorie intake should come from natural or added sugars.

Sugar is often thought of as empty calories or discretionary calories. Sugars are one of the major contributors to obesity, offering no nutritional value. However, sugar does provide temporary energy, which is often replaced with tiredness when it wears off. Sugar is also a very important consideration for those who have been diagnosed with diabetes or who have a family history of the disease.

To find out if a particular food is high in sugar, check the ingredient label. If sugar or one of its forms listed above are included in the first three ingredients, you know that it contains a high sugar content. Sugar sweetened cereal, candy, cakes, cookies, and drinks like cappuccino, soda pop and energy drinks are usually high in sugar. We expect those foods to contain sugar; but, sugar is included in non-sweet foods, as well—like canned spaghetti sauce and soups. So, if you're attempting to reduce your sugar intake, you should pay attention to the food labels of all food, not just sweets.

Glycerin: Glycerin or glycerol is similar to sugar in that it is used as a sweetener. It is also a solvent and added to foods to enhance preservation. Glycerin can be added to foods as a filler, as well as a thickening agent. Glycerol contains 27 calories per teaspoon, but is better for you than sugar because it doesn't affect blood sugar levels or contribute to tooth decay.

Also listed on nutrition labels are vitamin and mineral information and the percent of the daily recommended dosage contained in one serving. This information can be helpful in determining if you're getting adequate iron or calcium in your daily diet.

While we're talking about food labels, let's also take a look at some common categories used in marketing food and what they really mean.

- Reduced Sodium: While some people interpret this label to mean that a food is low in sodium, that isn't always the case. In order for a manufacturer to claim that food is "reduced," it must only reduce the original product's level of fat or sodium by 25%. This means that a food can still be quite high in sodium, but the percentage has been reduced from its original amount.

- Lower Fat or Reduced Fat: Like reduced sodium, this simply means that the product has 25% less fat in it than the original version. In other words, it could still be high in fat!

- Reduced Sugar: Like sodium and fat, reduced sugar refers to food or beverages which contain 25% less sugar than the original product.

- Sugar Free: Less than ½ gram of sugar per serving.

- No Fat or Fat Free: Foods that contain 0 to 0.5 grams of fat per serving, meaning some fat may be present.

- Low Fat: Unlike "lower or reduced" fat, low fat food contains less than 3 grams of fat in each serving.

- Low Calories: Contains 1/3 of the amount of calories contained in the original product.

- No calories / Calorie Free: Contains 0 to 5 calories per serving, so this label doesn't always mean zero calories.

- Low Sodium: 140 mgs or less of sodium per serving.

- Lite: Food claiming to be "lite" contains 50 percent less fat per serving from the original product, or it contains 1/3 of the calories of the original version.

- No salt or salt free: Each serving contains less than 5mgs of sodium.

- High Fiber: High fiber foods must contain 5 g or more per serving. High fiber food must also be low fat (less than 3 grams of fat per serving) or the total fat appears alongside the high fiber phrase on the label.

Take a trip through the grocery store and check out the nutrition labels for the foods you usually like to eat. Take your time, reading the labels to find out which foods are better for you and which aren't. While this diet doesn't measure fats, carbohydrates, cholesterol or sugar—just calories—it is in your best interest to know what you're eating. Because of my concern with high blood pressure and diabetes (it runs in my family) I've opted to eat less salt and sugar in my diet and when I do, I balance it out by eating some protein or fiber along with it to keep it from spiking my insulin. I was surprised that some foods which I believed were good for me were very bad for my diet, while others were surprisingly low in calories and could be incorporated into my daily plan very easily.

Chapter Twenty-One

GOT WATER?

Like the many ads touting the benefits of drinking milk, a dieter also has a faithful companion that will provide abundant results—water. Water is truly the one greatest natural appetite suppressant available on the market!

But, that only scratches the surface of the benefits a dieter receives from a cool, refreshing glass of water. Water has zero calories, and it tastes great! It goes with everything and is readily available when you want it, either straight from the tap or in a convenient bottle.

The real benefits of water are enjoyed after drinking it. As much as 75 percent of our body is made up of water, including our muscles, organs, bones and skin. It's a vital ingredient in keeping the awesome machine called the human body working at its best. It's often been said that when dieter's first lose weight, it is mostly water weight. So, you might think that we shouldn't replace that weight, but that's wrong! The more water we drink, the faster we'll lose weight! The reason for that is because water flushes fat and toxins from our body, helping our organs to digest and metabolize the food we do eat. No other food or liquid can claim to do the same. Coffee, tea, soda pop and juice are fluids which we often enjoy, but they too often introduce caffeine (a diuretic which further dehydrates the body) and sugar, and we know that sugar isn't good for weight loss. Water is the sole source of natural hydration that the body craves.

When you're craving food or feeling a hunger pang, have a glass of water. You might not be hungry at all, but simply craving the hydration you need from clean, pure water. An eight ounce glass of water will fill your stomach, sending it signals that it's full, tiding you over until snack or meal time. It's so effective in curbing the appetite that it's recommended that we consume at least 64 ounces of water each and every day!

To put it simply, water is the mainstay of our bodies. There would be no life without it. While it keeps our bodies functioning and performing their best, it also curbs our appetite, nourishes our skin, flushes out toxins, and speeds up metabolism! It builds our muscles, trims away our fat, and gives us a secret weapon to fight off hunger attacks. So, whether you're at home or on the go, grab a glass of H_2O for a convenient and inexpensive boost to your health. Your body will thank you in so many ways as you quench your thirst and melt the pounds away.

Chapter Twenty-Two

IS INSULIN GUILTY OR INNOCENT IN WEIGHT GAIN?

When talking about insulin levels, most people believe that assume that any reference to insulin is in regard to conditions like high or low blood sugar. In a manner of speaking, that is correct, but insulin plays a larger role in our weight than determining whether we are victims of diseases related to high or low blood sugar.

I've learned through the years that insulin is one of the reasons why my body doesn't want to burn excess fat. The calorie counting diet I support works if my body uses more calories than it takes in. But there's one glitch that can throw it all askew—Insulin. Insulin can be guilty of preventing the body from burning fat, rather than helping it to do so.

Before I explain how insulin and fat are related, I want to remind you that if you have diabetes or a blood sugar condition or disease, it is imperative that you see a doctor before you begin any weight loss program. This is far too important not to stress one more time!

That said, let's look at an example of how insulin prevents us from losing fat and can be responsible for making us store even more fat!

Sally is on a diet. She's conscientious at all times, watching her caloric intake, eating foods which are nutritious and healthy, and even taking the time to workout at the gym three or four times a week. But, Sally can't seem to lose weight. Her body fat levels are the same as they were before she started her diet and fitness plan. What is she doing wrong?

Sally is doing a lot of things right, but she's not taking her insulin levels into consideration. Insulin helps regulate the amount of sugar in our blood and keeps many of our organs functioning properly. When the blood has too much sugar, insulin works to bring it back down. Insulin is a hormone, but not everyone knows that when their body has too much insulin, they store more fat! Every time we eat sugar, our body produces more insulin to bring our blood sugar down to acceptable levels. However, when our blood sugar and insulin levels rise, our body falsely believes that it has more than enough energy, so instead of using the calories we consume as energy, it stores them in the form of fat cells.

Even people who eat healthy foods and stay away from sweets suffer from the fat-storing effects of the body's insulin. Carbohydrates also trigger insulin production. Eating foods with white flour like bread, bagels, and rolls, can cause insulin levels to skyrocket, as will eating a lot of white rice and pasta. These foods metabolize quickly, as well, causing a fairly quick spike in insulin levels.

High levels of insulin store fat and prevent your body from burning excess fat. Therefore, Sally in the example above can diet and exercise, doing all the right things, but still not obtain the weight loss she's working so very hard for. In that instance, Sally would have to pay attention to her insulin levels, reducing bad carbs like white flour, pasta, and rice, as well as sugar, to keep her insulin levels low enough that her body will begin to burn fat, not store it.

Sally might also want to take a close look at how much processed foods she eats. Processed foods are also guilty for increasing insulin levels because in preparation, the nutritional value is lessened and the carbs are refined, causing them to metabolize even faster. Processed foods also cause further damage by adding sugars and even trans fat to the original product. As a result, some processed foods can cause a significant increase in the body's insulin production, which in turn affects metabolism, causing food to metabolize faster or slower.

Apart from avoiding white sugar and flour-based foods, what can you do? It's been recommended that when you are eating food high in refined carbohydrates that you add a little fat or protein, which slow down the speed that carbs are absorbed by the body. It's really not complicated. If you want toast, spread a pat of butter or margarine on it or include a little peanut butter on your bagel.

Sally and dieters like her will have faster results by controlling the amount of insulin their body produces. By consuming fewer carbohydrates and sugar, they'll also control the amount of insulin in their body, which is not only guilty of making them fat, but keeping them there.

Chapter Twenty-Three

SUGAR VERSUS INSULIN

You can fool some of the people some of the time, but when it comes to sugar, you can't fool your body. One of the first things most people do when they diet is to cut back on their sugar intake. They buy sugar-free cookies, cakes, candy, and soda pop, thinking they can still have the sweet treats their body craves, without the extra calories. They purchase boxes of artificial sweeteners for their coffee, tea, cereal or grapefruit to mimic the flavor of sugar while keeping it low in calories. Sounds like a plan, right?

Wrong. When you choose some artificial sweeteners over natural ones, your body can't be tricked as easily as your taste buds. Lab studies have shown that the body does know the difference. In fact, animals who were given artificial sweeteners ate more than animals who were given the same foods sweetened with natural sugars. Not only did they eat more, but they consumed more calories, as well. As a result, the animals who consumed natural sugars, like glucose, actually weighed less than those who were given foods sweetened with non-caloric or low-calories additives.

It seems that our bodies are smarter than we think they are. When we anticipate a sweet treat, our body immediately understands that it's going to have to burn more calories, so it responds by boosting our metabolism. However, when we eat foods sweetened with low or no-calorie substitutes, the body doesn't get that boost and our metabolism drops. When that happens, the result is opposite of what we expect—the body stores the calories it does get for future use, rather than burning them!

It could be the result of our programming or our chemistry. Regardless, the end result of eating food which has been sweetened with artificial sweeteners (which our body can't use in balancing insulin) seems to be that we tend to eat more food to compensate for what we know we aren't getting! The body knows what fuel we give it, and it's also aware of what fuels it's missing. Therefore, depriving your body totally of the calories natural sugars doesn't always work because it will try to make up for it by demanding an extra serving of something later in the day.

Diet pop is another culprit. Rather than helping us lose weight, studies have found that it actually increases the chance that we'll be overweight! This is proof that our bodies don't always respond to our weight loss efforts like we want them to. In addition, diet pop and other food and drinks sweetened with artificial low-calorie sweeteners can heighten the likelihood of developing insulin resistance. Insulin is responsible for regulating the sugar in our blood and contributes greatly to the function of many of our organs.

Is it worth confusing your body to sacrifice 15 calories? That's how many calories are in one teaspoon of sugar. To add insult to injury, there is a lot we don't know about artificial sweeteners, including long-term side effects and how safe they are to consume. While one study might show that there are no "known" side effects, another might indicate a multitude of potential problems they can cause.

But yet, we know that sugar isn't always good for us, either. What's the answer? I believe it might just be that we eat sugars (granulated, powdered, brown sugar, etc.) in moderation. In that way, we give the body what it needs to boost our metabolism, without giving it excess calories which would result in weight gain. For those times when we want something sweet, there are other natural sugars available which can provide the flavor we crave and the metabolic rate we want in a lower calorie sweetener.

While we're learning that sugar substitutes can make us fat, we're learning more about alternate natural sugars which don't. As people find that artificial sweeteners don't provide the same flavor and satisfaction as their beloved natural sugars, they're seeking alternate substitutes which offer better flavor and fewer health concerns.

Welcome Agave and Stevia to the sweet team. Both of these sugar substitutes are derived from natural, not artificial, means and they offer a tempting, yet healthy, alternative to the bitter taste left behind by artificial sweeteners.

Agave: A natural nectar, Agave is derived from fructose, which comes from fruits and vegetables. It's actually sweeter than the refined sugars we're used to eating, but it's healthier. Agave has a lower glycemic index than sugar; therefore, it's less likely to escalate fat storage in the body, welcome news for any dieter. This is one reason that Agave is preferred by people on low carbohydrate diets.

Agave also doesn't raise our blood sugar levels rapidly. This factor alone makes it a safe alternative to sugar because it is less likely to contribute to some diseases, like diabetes, high blood pressure or even abdominal weight gain. Although it is safer than sugar for diabetics, it should be used in moderation since it does include fructose. But, its supporters contend that even for diabetics, it's a welcome alternative to other sweeteners which can spike blood sugar rapidly. Of course, the use of any sugar or sweetener by a person with diabetes should be first approved by his or her physician.

If there is one downside to Agave, it's that it has more calories per unit than regular sugars. However, on the up side, it's reported to be 40 percent sweeter than sugar, so you would use far less to obtain the same level of sweetness.

Healthier than regular and refined sugars, Agave lends itself well as an ingredient in cooking, providing many of the same qualities as sugar, such as browning and thickening agents. But, it's also well known in some circles for its healing benefits, such as fighting bacteria. As a home remedy, it's used as a skin balm and a dressing for wounds.

So, while we can't forget that Agave does have calories, its low glycemic levels and the body's healthier response to it make it an attractive supplement to our daily diet.

Stevia: Stevia is an herb that's been used as a dietary supplement for years. It has absolutely no calories, no carbohydrates, and doesn't spike blood sugar levels. Stevia is much more potent than other sugars and artificial sweeteners, too.

Considered to be generally safe, the use of Stevia as a food additive is still being studied, but it's been determined that in high doses (as a supplement), it reduces blood pressure and glucose levels. That's good news for people with certain kinds of diabetes or hypertension. However, Stevia can actually make insulin perform better, so anyone with diabetes who uses Stevia is strongly urged to monitor their blood sugar levels very closely and seek the advice of their doctor.

New on the market for use as a sweetener, Stevia is already being used in beverages and is available as a sugar substitute. It's predicted that it will soon be approved for even wider use as an ingredient in food products and drinks

While these alternatives to sugar and artificial sweeteners are appealing to those who want to keep their blood sugar levels in check, there are other things you can do which will contribute greatly to your efforts:

- Eat every three to four hours will keep your blood sugar levels from spiking immediately after eating, then dropping to extremely low levels when you're hungry.

- Eat breakfast every day. This will help you get your blood sugar levels to a normal range at the beginning of the day, which will make it easier to regulate.

- Snack between meals to quell cravings for sweets. Choose snacks rich in protein and fiber. Fruits and vegetables are always good choices.

- Increase your daily intake of fiber, which will not only keep you regulated, but it also slows the release of sugar into the blood stream. Foods high in fiber include fruits, vegetables, whole grains, and nuts.

- Exercise! Even taking a walk every day will help you keep those blood sugar levels under control.

By choosing a diet high in protein, you'll reduce your cravings for carbohydrates. Those carbs are usually very high in sugar. Protein also helps you feel full for a longer period of time, reducing the likelihood that you'll be reaching for a sweet snack too soon after eating.

Fiber, on the other hand, plays a big role in the release of sugar into the bloodstream, keeping it continuous, rather than at extreme highs and lows. Adding more fiber to your diet will help prevent symptoms like headaches, nervousness, and nausea, which are a few symptoms of low blood sugar.

As you can see, what you eat does matter. By choosing natural sweeteners as a healthier alternative to refined sugar and artificial sweeteners, you can reduce your caloric intake, lower your glycemic levels, and regulate your blood sugar in a healthy manner. By bumping up the fiber and protein in your daily diet and supplementing that with daily exercise, you can help your body regulate your blood sugar levels, keeping them under control. Not only with you feel better, but you'll be less apt to overeat or snack throughout the day. It's the natural way to diet and be healthy!

Chapter Twenty-Four

TO EXERCISE—OR NOT?

Weight gain is caused by taking in more calories than we use in our daily life. When the calories exceed what we burn, they are stored by our body as fat. So, is the answer to reduce the number of calories we intake, increase the calories we burn, or both?

I told you earlier that I chose a sedentary lifestyle when I determined the daily calorie intake I needed to get down to my desired weight. While I'm not always sedentary, I've found that this method works best for me for several reasons.

First, I wanted to make sure I lost weight, but in a healthy way. My intention was to make weight loss my priority. By choosing a sedentary or less active lifestyle, I'm guaranteeing that the calories I'm allowed will result in weight loss, regardless if I'm physically active or not. It was important to me to eliminate any room for error, and I know that there are days when I'm more active than others. I wanted my diet to work *every* day!

In addition, in the past, I've found that diets are hard to incorporate into my life. I'm a wife and a mother; I'm also active in the community. As a result, sometimes it's more than a little difficult for me to schedule a block of time specifically for exercising. So, I chose first to focus on the calories I consume and the weight loss, hoping as soon as those results were visible, I'd find it easier to exercise and be more motivated to do so.

I was right! The calorie count for a sedentary life provided me with a greater guarantee of weight loss, and at a faster pace. I was able to focus my time and energy on the foods I ate, journaling my diet, and retraining my body to become more aware of when I'm full, hungry, or bored.

If you're already physically active or go to the gym on a regular basis, great! I encourage you to keep up the good work. It will help you burn more calories and make your weight loss faster. However, for people like me, who haven't been as physically active in the past, introducing a new exercise program into a busy life at the same time we're trying to shed extra weight can be a challenge. In dieting, the fewer challenges, the better!

Losing weight has its advantages. Not only do we look better, we feel better, also. After losing 15 pounds, I've found that I have more energy and feel healthier than I did before. Each pound is another incentive to meet my goal, and that's a great reason to begin incorporating exercise into my daily routine. Being a few pounds lighter makes physical activity easier and less strenuous, too. The extra energy I've gotten makes me *want* to talk a brisk walk, rather than having to! When exercise is a chore, it's as bad as housework. You'll put it off as long as possible!

When you begin your exercise program, don't overdo it right away. Start small and increase your increments as you become more comfortable. One of the downfalls for many dieters is that they start a diet and an exercise program at the same time, not realizing that muscle weighs more than fat. So, as they're losing fat, they're actually gaining some of their weight back in increased muscle weight. Then, they become discouraged because the needle on the scale isn't moving fast enough. I've found that I have more motivation to follow my diet when I can see and measure real progress, and then incorporate an exercise plan into it.

I've learned that even sedentary people can ease exercise into their life without a lot of effort, sweat or huffing and puffing. This works for people who are homebound or have a desk job, too. While you're sitting, you can flex and tone your muscles, your legs, thighs and buns. Tighten, hold, release. There are many exercises which are designed to tone different areas of the body. Here are a few:

1. While you're sitting (watching television, browsing the Internet, or sitting at your desk), tighten your buttocks, holding for a count of ten, then release. Repeat ten times. Then alternate, tightening your left bun only for ten seconds, then the right.

2. Leg Lifts: While you're sitting at your desk or in a chair, raise one leg off the floor, straightening the knee. Use your thigh to raise and lower your leg (without touching the floor at the bottom) and repeat ten times with each leg.

3. Side benders. In a sitting position with your spine straight, bend sideways at the waist, dipping down as far as you can (don't fall off your chair!) and return to a straight position. Repeat on other side. Do as many reps as you feel comfortable doing to help tone your waistline.

These exercises and others can be incorporated into your day by doing them when you're talking on the phone, folding laundry, making dinner, or washing dishes. Before long, you'll catch yourself doing them without even knowing it!

You can also increase your physical activity by changing your routine in small ways so that you burn more calories. Don't choose the closest parking spot to the mall entrance, making it necessary to walk just a little further. You can also choose the heart healthy way and take the stairs instead of the elevator. Other ways to get yourself moving can be as easy as putting the remote control across the room so you have to get up to turn the channel.

There is an exercise program for everyone, and it's important that at some point in your weight-loss program, you incorporate it into your life. You'll look better, feel better, and be healthier when you do! Regardless of what type of activity or exercise you do, get in the habit of charting it so you can see and gauge your progress. I've developed a basic exercise log you can use to keep track of your physical fitness activities. Feel free to use the chart on the following page or download the one on my website at www.suzonneunderwood.com.

WEEKLY EXERCISE LOG			
DATE		TIME SPENT	CALORIES BURNED

Chapter Twenty-Five

WALK IT OFF

There are so many ways to whittle the waist, tone muscles, and become physically fit, and there are just as many exercise machines and programs to work each area of the body. Some machines mimic bikes, stairs, and walking, while others build strength through the use of resistance. These machines can be accessed by purchasing them, or becoming a member at a gym, fitness center, or weight loss club. Buying one or more can be an expensive investment, and when we do, too often we don't have space to store them or we lose interest and they become dust collectors or clothes hangers. Memberships in a fitness center or gym require scheduling the time for the workout, driving to and from the gym, and, for some, day care for children. I know how hard it is to find an effective exercise program that works, is convenient, and is also one that I can and will religiously follow.

That's why I've become a fan of walking. Walking for fitness or weight loss is an excellent exercise. For one thing, it's free. There's no cost or obligation to participate! God gave us the necessary equipment, so we don't have to purchase any, and we can walk whenever we want, for as long as we want, wherever we want. It doesn't matter if we're already fit or if we are sedentary, and walking doesn't discriminate between those who are young, old, rich, poor, thin or heavy. I see walking as a one size fits all exercise plan!

Walking is something everyone can do. It isn't strenuous and is less likely to cause physical injury than most other cardiovascular exercises, such as running or jogging. That's because walking is a low impact form of exercise, which doesn't jar our joints. Therefore, there are few side effects from walking, and any side effects one might encounter are usually minor and short-term.

Above all, walking is convenient. I can decide when and where I choose to walk and how long I want to walk. I don't have to worry about open times at the gym or traffic. The only thing that impedes my ability to walk at will is the weather and my own schedule. Choosing walking over any other exercise is the most flexible option. If I wish, I can walk in the early morning hours and observe my world as its waking up, or I can wait until the kids go to school so I can walk without other demands on my time. On the other hand, I might choose an afternoon or evening walk, asking my daughters to join me. While it is exercise, it's also a great way to spend time together, get fresh air, and enjoy nature and my surroundings.

But, perhaps those aren't even the greatest benefits of walking. Walking burns calories, which promotes weight loss. It tones many muscle groups and provides a cardiovascular workout which is gentle on, but very beneficial, to the heart. When you learn the many health benefits gained from walking, I hope you'll also be encouraged to take up the sport.

- Walking burns calories, which helps speed weight loss. It's also a great exercise for maintaining weight.

- Walking is physical exercise, which does help curb hunger!

- Because walking is credited with weight loss and weight control, it's very beneficial to overall physical health. A daily habit of walking can:
  - **Reduce blood pressure.** The heart is a muscle, and physical activity strengthens the muscle, making its job easier. A strong heart requires less work to pump blood, which puts less pressure on the arteries which feed it to our other organs.
  - **Lower the risk of heart disease.** For the same reasons that walking reduces blood pressure, it also helps to prevent heart disease. In addition, physical activity reduces the LDL or bad cholesterol in our blood, which builds plaque in our arteries and can cause a heart attack.
  - **Reduce the risk of obtaining Type 2 Diabetes.** Combined with even a small amount of weight loss and reduced fat intake, walking can reduce the risk of Type 2 diabetes.
  - **Reduce the risk of stroke.** Daily walking can lower the risk of stroke by as much as 50 percent.
  - **Prevent gallstones.** Yes, daily walking has even been credited with reducing the need for gallstone surgery!
  - **Strengthening bones and joints.** Regular walking helps our bones maintain their strength and density, while also keeping joints, like hips, limber and flexible.
  - **Prevent certain cancers.** Walking and other forms of physical activity are one source of preventive maintenance in reducing the risk of breast and colon cancers.

- o **Reducing pain from arthritis.** Pain from back problems and arthritis can be lowered for those who take a brisk walk every day.

- o **Improve sleep.** Walking and other forms of physical activity help produce a good night's sleep and are even responsible for improving some instances of sleep apnea.

- o **Reduce stress.** Walking is easy to do, and it's also calming. It reduces anxiety and stress, which we all know can be the culprit of nervous snacking!

As you can see, walking is great preventive medicine! It's a non-strenuous, low impact exercise that delivers so many benefits, not only in weight loss, but in our overall health and life. While side effects are rare, you can do your part to eliminate them by:

- Consulting with a physician before you start any exercise program. Your doctor can provide you with limits and guidelines appropriate for your fitness level and body. Following those guidelines will prevent you from too much exertion or stress.

- Buy a good pair of walking shoes. Minor aches are one of the side effects of walking. Shoes with proper arch and ankle support, cushion and soles will reduce the strain on ankles, feet, hips, and even your back. Look for shoes which are properly vented, allowing your feet to breathe and stay dry.

- Walk at a pace which is comfortable for you. If you cannot walk at a brisk pace for an extended period, switch between regular walking and brisk walking. A good guide to follow is your breathing: if you're breathing very easy, you can probably step up the pace. However, if you're out of breath, it's time to slow down for a while. Another good gauge for setting your pace is to keep your walking at a pace where you can still make conversation.

- If you're going to do some brisk walking, consider a few stretching exercises to get your muscles warmed up. Proper stretching prevents injuries.

- To reduce the impact on your feet, make sure the heel hits the pavement or surface first, then roll the foot forward to the toes. Walking is low impact; however, the harder the surface under your feet, the more impact there will be. Concrete and asphalt are used on sidewalks, roads, and walking paths and they are safe, even surfaces for walking. Walking trails might also be made of lower softer materials, like mulched bark, a gravel/dust mixture, or even sawdust.

- If you walk at night, wear reflective clothing and carry a flashlight. Consider walking with a buddy!

To get maximum benefits from walking, you need to be diligent. You need to commit to a steady and regular walking program. If you're not physically fit or haven't exercised in some time, start out with slow and regular walking. As you become more comfortable, you can increase your pace and incorporate brisk walking. After you've mastered that, you might want to try power walking for a more strenuous workout. To determine speed, consider 2.0 mph a slow, leisurely stroll, and 5.0 mph to be a maximum high-speed brisk walk. You know you're walking at a good steady pace when you hit speeds of 3 to 4 miles per hour.

How much and how often should you walk? That's up to you and how comfortable you are, but take into consideration that the best benefits are derived when you walk 5 days a week, for 30 minutes each day. You can break that up, if you want, walking for 15 minutes during your lunch hour, and another 15 minutes around the block after dinner.

Now, I know you've been wondering just how many calories you'll burn by walking. Each person is different, and it depends on their current weight, pace, and walking location, i.e., is the surface flat, on an incline, are there stairs? The formula below will give you an idea how many calories you can expect to burn per each mile walked at a pace of 3 miles per hour.

Multiply .63 x your weight = Calories burned per mile

For example, if you weigh 150 pounds, you'd burn about 95 calories per mile.

At that rate, walking burns almost as many calories as running or jogging, and it's easier on the muscles, joints, and heart. It's also an exercise you can enjoy year round. If it's raining, grab an umbrella or go to the mall, where you might find a group of fellow walkers who are on the same quest you are—to lose weight and become more fit so you can enjoy a longer, healthier life.

Like me, you might even find that you enjoy walking so much that you start to forget that it's exercise at all!

Chapter Twenty-Six

TIPS AND TRICKS TO CURB YOUR APPETITE AND AVOID TEMPTATION

There's no doubt about it. Every dieter encounters temptation once in a while—it's part of the package. While we can occasionally indulge in a treat, sometimes, it's better for us if we avoid it completely. Here are some tips and tricks I've found which will curb your appetite and keep you from feeling guilty afterward.

- Drink water. Drink plenty of water throughout the day to replenish and cleanse your body. An 8 to 10 ounce glass or bottle of water will also keep your stomach from feeling empty.

- Counter a sweet craving with the opposite. The next time you have an urge for chocolate, eat a dill pickle! Really, it works! The sour note of the pickle will overwhelm any desire for sugar or sweets. (And a pickle has a lot fewer calories!)

- When you know that you really want a snack that's not good for you, brush your teeth! That just-brushed-feeling (and taste) will help you say no.

- Substitute low-fat spray butter for traditional butter or margarine. You'll use a lot less and it has fewer calories, as well.

- You can have popcorn while you're dieting. Actually, popcorn is a high fiber food which is good for you—as long as you don't pour butter all over it. Try flavored sprinkle cheeses, instead.

- Suck on sugar-free hard candy as an alternative to munching on crunchy snacks.

- Drink ginger ale or tonic water with a twist of lemon or lime as an alternative to fattening wine or alcohol at parties.

- Whole grains are healthier alternatives to white bread and flour, which have less nutritional value and are more fattening.

- Freeze grapes for an easy and refreshing sweet treat. You can pop them in your mouth frozen or thawed.

- Freeze your own popsicles, made from natural 100% juices, for a healthy and sweet snack.

- Eat dry cereal (minus the milk) as an easy, crunchy snack. Cereal is vitamin enhanced and easy to measure and pre-pack for a snack on the go.

- Put your blender or food processor to good use and make your own applesauce, adding spices like cinnamon and nutmeg instead of sugar for a flavorful treat.

- Baked apples or pears are also a great dessert, once again adding cinnamon or nutmeg to add new life to a favorite food.

- Sunflower seeds are a great way to make a snack last a long time, because you have to work to get them out of their outer shell!

- Have a vegetarian dinner at least one night a week. There are so many different things you can do with vegetables that you won't miss having meat or fried foods at all.

- Put your fork down between bites. It is true that we eat too fast! Putting your fork down gives you a chance to thoroughly chew and enjoy your food. In addition, because it takes longer for you to eat when you do, you'll know when you're full before you overeat.

- Learn to eat when you're hungry. Even something little will keep you from cheating later.

- Take inventory of your refrigerator. Substitute lower calorie dressings, mayonnaise, lunch meat, milk, cheese, and yogurt for their higher-calorie counterparts.

- Don't eat after 8 pm. Your body won't have a chance to naturally burn and metabolize your food and you'll get a better night's sleep!

- Substitute higher calorie meats with lower fat meat, poultry, and fish. Prepare meat in healthier ways, avoiding the frying pan and choosing instead to grill or broil food.

These are just some of the tips you can use to curb your appetite and to stay on track and focused on your goal! Remember, keep your eye on the prize and you'll reap the rewards!

Chapter Twenty-Seven

A SNACK A DAY CAN HELP
KEEP THE POUNDS AWAY

Snacking is a major source of hidden calories in our diets. The reason for this is because the foods we choose to snack on are usually high in calories for a relatively small portion. Because of that, when we snack, we often don't curb our hunger or satisfy our cravings. Then, we're left with a desire to eat even more.

I think snacks play a very important role in our diets. Rather than eliminate them, I turn to snacks to keep me on track. That's why I like to make wise snack choices, ones which will actually satisfy my hunger and hold me over until the next meal, provide me with energy, and which have some nutritional value.

A good snack will curb your hunger and provide you with some nutrition. One of the main reasons we snack is for energy, so if you're in need of a pick-me-up, avoid snacks like soda or candy and anything which has a lot of sugar (carbohydrates). Instead, select whole-grains, unsweetened cereals, cheese, yogurt or peanut butter. Nuts are a good source of protein, as well, but avoid any with added salt or sugars or nuts which have a high level of fat. A protein rich snack will give you the boost of energy you need to get you through until your next meal.

WEIGHT-LOSS SNACKS

Calories	Food Choices
10 calories	1 large stalk of celery 2 dill pickles
25-30 calories	1 cup raw vegetables 6 medium baby carrots 1 cup cherry tomatoes
60 calories	2 cups air-popped or light popcorn 1 cup of cantaloupe or grapes 1 small can of vegetable juice 1 mandarin orange
80 calories	8 ounces of skim milk Sun Maid Fruit Bits, ¼ cup Del Monte Fruit & Nut Snacks (comes in snack packs) Cranberry Medley 1 Luna Mini Protein Bar 1 Jell-O Sugar Free Chocolate Pudding Snack with five strawberries
100 calories	1 cup sliced bananas and fresh raspberries 2 domino-sized slices low-fat Colby or cheddar cheese 1 fat-free chocolate pudding cup 1.5 ounces of dried fruit 1 medium apple 1 banana 3 ounces of tuna packed in water (not oil), no mayonnaise 1 Slim Fast Chocolate Caramel Snack Bar 1 Slim Fast Protein Snack Chew 8 ounces of 1% milk
120 calories	8 ounces of 2% milk 3 pretzel rods 7 reduced fat Triscuit wafers 1 can Del Monte Fruit Pleasures Bite Size Delights Raspberry Flavored Peaches ¾ cup Apple Cinnamon Cheerios (no milk) 3/4 cup Cinnamon Life (no milk)
150 calories	1/2 cup frozen, low-fat yogurt topped with 1/2 cup blueberries

	1 cup sliced apples with 1 tablespoon smooth peanut butter
	4 rye crackers
	20 to 22 raw almonds
	7 ounces of grapes
	8 ounces of whole milk
200 calories	1/4 cup dry roasted soy nuts (calories vary by brand)
	1/3 cup granola
	1 cup low-fat cottage cheese topped with 1/2 cup sliced fresh peaches
	1 Slim Fast Shake

Some food values obtained from: Department of Agriculture — Nutrient Data Laboratory, 2007

Those are great ideas for those who prefer to eat fresh fruit and vegetables, as well as for those who don't mind measuring and prepackaging snacks. If you're like me, though, you'll enjoy the convenience of individually wrapped servings of snacks which are available in stores. They take the guesswork out of your diet with no need to measure, divide, or weigh your food. In addition, individually wrapped prepackaged snacks usually don't require cooking or utensils and are easy to open and eat with little mess or fuss.

For those with a sweet tooth, Hostess makes a line of 100 calorie snacks, like mini blueberry muffins. Other food manufacturers who offer 100 calorie prepackaged snacks include:

Nabisco: Ritz Snack Mix, Cheese Nips crackers, Wheat Thins, Honey Maid Grahams, Chips Ahoy Thin Crisps, Oreo Thin Crisps, Planters Peanut Butter Crisps, Mr. Salty Chocolate Covered Pretzels, 100 calorie Mixed Berry Fruit Snacks, 100 calorie Chewy Granola Bars

<u>Doritos</u>: Nacho Cheese Flavored Tortilla Chips, Cool Ranch Flavored Tortilla Chips

<u>General Mills</u>: Pop Secret Kettle Corn

<u>Pringles</u> 100 calorie packs

<u>Quaker Oats</u> Caramel Corn Rice Cakes

<u>Thomas'</u> Light Multi-Grain English Muffin

<u>Frito Lay</u>: SUNCHIPS Harvest Cheddar Flavored Multigrain Snacks or Cheetos Crunchy Mini Bites

As you can see, there is a large variety of flavors and foods from which you can choose. From fresh fruit and vegetables to nuts and whole grains, there are textures and tastes to fit everyone. I have my favorite snacks, but I also try to add variety to keep myself from getting bored with them. I also try to choose snacks which provide nutritional value and other benefits, like fiber, so my snacks are nutritious, as well as satisfying.

WAIT!
I WANT TO HEAR FROM YOU!

Nobody looks forward to dieting, but I think we all look forward to finding a diet that really works—one which delivers exactly what it promises. That's why I wanted to share my weight loss strategy with you. In my quest to drop pounds, I've found a way that does work and it will keep on working as long as I follow it. The added bonus is that it is not only a diet, but a maintenance plan, as well, which will keep me from regaining my weight once I've met my goal. I've chosen this diet because it's not temporary, but rather a permanent change in my eating habits which will promote a slimmer, trimmer body and a healthier lifestyle.

Because diets carry a stigma of being an inconvenience in our lives, I've tried to include as much information in this book as possible, from ways to get motivated and stay there, to my weight loss tips and tricks. I've provided information on effective, yet easy and enjoyable, exercise to help you get moving, as well. To make it even easier for you, I hope you refer to the snack calorie chart as you're planning your own menus. I hope that you find the benefit in convenient, prepackaged foods, so you spend less time planning, cooking, and cleaning and more time doing the things you enjoy.

An informed dieter makes the very best choices. I encourage you to visit the websites listed at the end of this book for useful online information, tools, charts, resources, and articles. As you weigh your options, I encourage you to join groups, visit websites and share your diet tips and tricks with others. To that end, I invite you to visit me at www.suzonneunderwood.com and share with me your progress. Let me know what works for you and what doesn't; share the tips and strategies you've learned during your journey to a new, trimmer you! You've got the tools and the motivation to use them. I wish you much success and happy dieting!

About the Author

SUZONNE EVANS UNDERWOOD

Suzonne Evans Underwood and her husband, Bobby, reside in Monroe, Louisiana, with their two daughters. Suzonne has a love for reading, writing, decorating, and antiques. She enjoys cooking and entertaining, fundraising, Bible study and spending time with family and friends. Suzonne is also actively involved in her children's schools, church, and community functions.

Suzonne invites her readers to visit her website: www.SuzonneUnderwood.com where they can share their experiences in her blog and access articles, news, and updated information to assist them in making healthier and more creative choices.

PLACES TO GO – THINGS TO SEE

Find out what you'll look like before and after losing weight with this free online weight loss simulator!
http://www.prevention.com/mvm/main.html

Daily Calorie Counter: Find out how much you should eat to maintain your weight:
http://www.prevention.com/cda/toolfinder.do?tf_type=calorie_calculator&channel=weight.loss&cm_mmc=Mag_URL-_-2007_November-_-Weight%20Loss-_-Calorie%20Calculator

Free Online Diet and Exercise Journal: http://www.my-calorie-counter.com/

Free Diet and Weight Loss Journal: www.fitday.com

Exercise Calorie Counter (Find out how many calories you burn in different exercise programs and workouts):
http://www.my-calorie-counter.com/

CalorieLab.com: Find the calorie count of 70,000 foods and 500 restaurant menus:
http://calorielab.com/index.html

CalorieSmart, an electronic pocket calorie calculator with a database of 35,000 foods and 250 restaurants.
http://www.fitsugar.com/74478

Doctor's Pocket Calorie, Fat, & Carbohydrate Counter: Plus 150 Fast Food Chains & Restaurants by Allan Borushek available at:

http://www.alibris.com/search/books/qwork/7810763/

Free Online Diet Plan, Fitness Tools and Support:
www.sparkpeople.com

Get inspired by reading other diet and exercise success
stories at:
http://www.shapefit.com/success-stories.html

Suggested Reading to Keep Motivated:
http://weightloss.about.com/od/weightloss101/a/101lesson
10.htm

Weight Loss Motivation and Tips:
http://www.fitnessmagazine.com/weight-
loss/tips/motivation/

Best Tips to Lose Weight – Free Healthy Weight Loss
Tips: http://www.weight-loss-health.com.au/
weight_loss_tips.htm

Articles by Weight Loss Coaches:
http://www.prevention.com/cda/categorypage.do?channel
=weight.loss&category=weight.loss.coaches

How to Find a Weight Loss Coach:
http://www.ehow.com/how_2125046_find-weight-loss-
coach.html?ref=fuel&utm_source=yahoo&utm_medium=s
sp&utm_campaign=yssp_art

Real Advice from a Weight Loss Coach:
http://www.weight-loss-consultant.com/

Printable Shopping List for Dieters:
http://www.gettinglean.com/shoplist.htm
Grocery List Generator and Nutrition Plans based on the
foods you like and your weight loss goals:
http://www.smartdiets.com/signup/index_blue.html

Slim-Fast® Plan, Activities, and Support:
www.slimfast.com

Personal Training Free and Online Exercise Routines &
Fast Weight Loss Diet Plans: www.freetrainers.com

Free Guide to Diet Plans, Menus, and Free Samples:
www.freedieting.com

Diet Tracker, Menus, Fitness Plans, etc.:
www.dietwatch.com

Recipes, Calorie Analyzers, Forums, Fast Food Info, and
Diet Secrets: www.freeweightloss.com

Free Calorie Counter, Weight Loss Calculators, and
Weight Loss Tutorial:
www.caloriesperhour.com

The Cambridge Diet Plans Foods for Life Nutritional
Supplements, low-calorie supplements that contain 100%
of recommended daily vitamins and nutrients:
http://www.sndi.biz/SNDI_clients/Suzonne-
Cambridge/cambridge-design.html

RESOURCES:

Insulin Resistance: Confused about carbohydrates? A quick guide to the carb spectrum by Marcelle Pick, OB/GYN   www.womentowomen.com/insulinresistance/carbohydratefoods.aspx

Body Recomposition: Insulin Levels and Fat Loss, http://www.bodyrecomposition.com/fat-loss/insulin-levels-and-fat-loss-qa.html

About.com Exercise, Rev Up Your Metabolism, Why food isn't the enemy by Paige Waehner, http://exercise.about.com/cs/weightloss/a/metabolism.htm

MedicineNet.com, Walking, Richard Weil, MEd, CDE, http://www.medicinenet.com/walking/article.htm

About.com: Walking, Benefits of Walking–How Walking Reduces Health Risks
http://walking.about.com/od/healthbenefits/Benefits_of_W alking_How_Walking_Reduces_Health_Risks.htm

Your Total Health Ideal Weight Calculator, http://dftools.ivillage.com/healthtools/calc_iw.cfm

Ideal Weights obtained from Metropolitan Life Insurance Company tables (1983)

American Cancer Society Calorie Counter: http://www.cancer.org/docroot/PED/content/PED_6_1x_C alorie_Calculator.asp
Department of Agriculture — Nutrient Data Laboratory, 2007

www.ingramcontent.com/pod-product-compliance
Lightning Source LLC
Chambersburg PA
CBHW071047290526
45795CB00004B/1362